PERSPECTIVES IN COGNITIVE NEUROSCIENCE
Stephen M. Kosslyn, *General Editor*

Printed in the United States of America

Second printing, 2002

First Harvard University Press paperback edition, 2002

Library of Congress Cataloging-in-Publication Data
Lieberman, Philip.
Human language and our reptilian brain : the subcortical bases of speech, syntax, and thought / Philip Lieberman.
p. cm.
Includes bibliographical references and index.
ISBN 0-674-00226-1 (cloth)
ISBN 0-674-00793-X (pbk.)
1. Neurolinguistics. 2. Basal ganglia. I. Title.
QP399.L535 2000
612.8'2—dc21 99-086092

Philip Lieberman

HUMAN LANGUAGE AND OUR REPTILIAN BRAIN

The Subcortical Bases of Speech, Syntax, and Thought

HARVARD UNIVERSITY PRESS
Cambridge, Massachusetts, and London, England

To Marcia, who did the impossible
for Lhakpa Dolma

Acknowledgments

Almost thirty years have passed since I proposed that the neural mechanisms that confer human syntactic ability evolved from ones originally adapted for motor control. In retrospect, my proposal was not original: Karl Lashley had come to a similar conclusion some twenty years earlier in a reference I had missed. Since then many people have provided experimental evidence and observations that support this theory. The insights provided by Paul MacLean's work offered a challenge to reconsider the role of our reptilian brain. My own efforts would not have been possible without my friend and colleague Joseph Friedman, who provided guidance concerning the nature of Parkinson's disease. Moreover, my research on the subcortical bases of speech, syntax, and thinking was enhanced through the participation of Allen Cymerman, Liane Feldman, Tecumseh Fitch, Jesse Hochstadt, Edward Kako, Erin Kuniholm, Hiroko Nakano, Emily Pickett, Athanassios Protopapas, Eric Reed, Chu-Yu Tseng, and Ted Young and many discussions with Sheila Blumstein, John Donoghue, Daniel Lieberman, and Emily, Hiroko, Jesse, Tecumseh, and Thanassi. Funds for much of the research that led to this book were provided by the National Aeronautics and Space Agency and the Federal Aviation Agency. And I owe special thanks to Elizabeth Bates, John Bradshaw, Fred Dick, John Donoghue, and Trevor Robbins, who reviewed and provided comments on earlier versions of this book. However, I probably would not have followed this line of inquiry if, in a year that now seems distant, Franklin Cooper and Alvin Liberman had not agreed to my attempting to answer a question, why apes don't talk, that seemingly was not related to the mandate of Haskins Laboratories. In Al's own words, but in a deeper evolutionary context, "speech is special."

Contents

Introduction *1*

1 Functional Neural Systems *19*

2 Speech Production and Perception *37*

3 The Lexicon and Working Memory *61*

4 The Subcortical Basal Ganglia *82*

5 The Evolution of the Functional Language System *124*

6 Commentary *157*

Notes *169*

References *181*

Index *209*

Figures

Figure I–1. Mesulam's network model of the neural bases of language 16
Figure 1–1. Lateral view of the left hemisphere of the human brain 21
Figure 1–2. A schematic multilayered network 26
Figure 1–3. Brodmann's maps of the cortical areas of the macaque monkey and human brains 28
Figure 2–1. The anatomy involved in the production of human speech 40
Figure 2–2. Two stylized formant frequency plots of [di] and [du] 50
Figure 2–3. Plots of averaged first and second formant frequencies of English vowels 52
Figure 2–4. "Naturalness" judgments of formant frequencies of synthesized English vowels 55
Figure 4–1. Basal ganglia of the human brain 84
Figure 4–2. General architecture of three basal ganglia circuits 86
Figure 4–3. Computational architecture of the basal ganglia 91
Figure 4–4. The Tower of London test array 114
Figure 4–5. Thinking time and number of perfect solutions on the Tower of London test 115
Figure 5–1. Head and neck of an adult male chimpanzee 137
Figure 5–2. Lateral view of an adult human supralaryngeal vocal tract 138

Figures

HUMAN LANGUAGE AND
OUR REPTILIAN BRAIN

Introduction

What are the brain bases of human language; how did they evolve? And what makes human language special?

For the past 200 years virtually all attempts to account for the neural bases and evolution of language have looked to the neocortex, the most recent evolutionary aspect of the mammalian brain. And in the past forty years, following Noam Chomsky's lead, linguistic research has virtually equated syntax with language; syntactic ability is taken to be a unique characteristic of the human mind deriving from an innate, genetically transmitted "instinct."

I shall attempt to shift the focus. The premise of this book is that language is not an instinct, based on genetically transmitted knowledge coded in a discrete cortical "language organ." Instead it is a learned skill, based on a functional language system (FLS) that is distributed over many parts of the human brain. The FLS regulates the comprehension and production of spoken language, which alone exists in no other living species. Moreover, the FLS is overlaid on sensorimotor systems that originally evolved to do other things and continue to do them now. Although the neural bases of language include the neocortex, some of the key structures of the FLS are subcortical basal ganglia—our reptilian brain. It too has evolved from its primeval reptilian form and, in concert with other structures of the brain, may be the key to human language and cognition.

The studies that I will discuss suggest that the FLS derives from mechanisms that yield timely motor responses to environmental challenges and opportunities—in short, motor activity that increases biological fitness, the survival of an individual's progeny. In this light, the subcortical basal ganglia structures usually associated with motor control that are key elements of the FLS reflect its evolutionary history—natural selection operated on neural mechanisms that yield adaptive, that is to say, "cognitive" motor responses in other species. And the basal ganglia, traditionally associated with reptilian brains (MacLean, 1973; Parent, 1986), derive from the brains of amphibians (Marin, Smeets, and Gonzalez, 1998). Ultimately, human linguistic and cognitive ability can be traced back to the learned motor responses of mollusks (Carew, Walters, and Kandel, 1981; Lieberman, 1984, pp. 57–78; 1991, pp. 123–124).

I also hope to show that though the neural substrate that allows us to acquire language is innate, we learn the sound pattern, words, and syntax of particular languages. Nor are the mental operations carried out by our brains compartmentalized in the manner proposed by most linguists and many cognitive scientists. The correct model for the functional organization of the human brain is not that offered by "modular" theorists such as Steven Pinker (1994, 1998)—a set of petty bureaucrats each of which controls a behavior and won't have anything to do with one another. The neural bases of human language are intertwined with other aspects of cognition, motor control, and emotion.

Neither the anatomy nor the physiology of the FLS can be specified with certainty given our current limited knowledge. The discussion here should be considered an outline and agenda for future research. However, converging behavioral and neurobiological data indicate that human language is regulated by a distributed network that includes subcortical structures, the traditional cortical "language" areas (Broca's and Wernicke's areas), and regions of the neocortex often associated with "nonlinguistic" aspects of cognition. As is the case for other neural systems, the architecture of the FLS consists of circuits linking segregated populations of neurons in neuroanatomical structures, cortical and subcortical, distributed throughout the brain. The FLS rapidly integrates sensory information with stored knowledge. The FLS is a dynamic system, enlisting additional neural resources in response to task difficulty. Regions of the frontal lobes of the human neocortex, implicated in abstract reasoning and planning (Goldstein, 1948; Mesulam, 1985; Stuss and Benson, 1986; Fuster, 1989; Grafman, 1989), and other cortical areas are recruited as task difficulty increases (Klein et al., 1994; Just et al., 1996).

In short, the human FLS is unique; no other living species possesses the neural capacity to command spoken language (or alternate manual systems), which serves as a medium for both communication and thought. However, its anatomy and physiology derive from neural structures and systems that regulate adaptive motor behavior in other animals. This evolutionary perspective may not be familiar to cognitive scientists, linguists, and perhaps some philosophers. But the insights gained by considering the probable evolutionary history of the FLS are of value to cognitive scientists and linguists as well as to neurobiologists. In time, "biological-linguists" working in an evolutionary framework will lead the way to new insights on the nature of language. Paraphrasing Dobzhansky, nothing in the biology of language makes sense except in the light of evolution.

Distributed Functional Neural Systems

The traditional view of the neural bases of complex behaviors derives from early nineteenth-century phrenology (Gall, 1809). Phrenologists claimed that different parts of the brain, which could be discerned by examining a person's cranium, were the "seats" of various aspects of behavior or character. Neophrenological theories do not claim that the bumps on a person's skull can tell you whether he is virtuous or can play the violin. Instead, they map complex behaviors to localized regions of the brain, on the assumption that a particular part of the brain regulates an aspect of behavior. Perhaps the best-known example is the traditional Broca-Wernicke model for the neural bases of human linguistic ability. Broca's 1861 study ascribed the expressive language deficits (word-finding difficulties and impediments in speech production) of a patient who had suffered a series of strokes to damage to "Broca's area," a frontal region of the neocortex. Shortly after, in 1874, "receptive" deficits in the comprehension of language were ascribed to damage to a posterior area of the cortex, "Wernicke's area." Lichtheim's 1885 model, subsequently restated by Geschwind (1970), claimed that the neurological basis of human language was a system linking Wernicke's area with Broca's area. According to this model, Wernicke's area processes incoming speech signals; information is then transmitted via a hypothetical cortical pathway to Broca's area, which serves as the "expressive" language output device. Subsequent research has shown that patients diagnosed as Broca's aphasics often produced sentences having simplified syntax and had difficulties comprehending distinctions in meaning conveyed by syntax (Zurif, Carramazza, and Meyerson, 1972). The Lichtheim-Geschwind theory is taken by linguists such as Chomsky (1986) and Pinker (1994) to be a valid model of the neural architecture underlying human linguistic ability. Pinker states: "Genuine language . . . is seated in the cerebral cortex, primarily the left perisylvian region" (1994, p. 334). He specifically identifies the "the human language areas . . . Wernicke's and Broca's areas and a band of fibers connecting the two" (p. 350). Many attempts to account for the evolution of human language (e.g., Williams and Wakefield, 1995; Harnad, personal communication; Calvin and Bickerton, 2000) do not question the validity of the Lichtheim-Geschwind model.

Although the Lichtheim-Geschwind model has the virtue of being simple, current neurophysiologic data show that it is wrong. Some regions of the neocortex are specialized to process particular stimuli, visual or auditory, while others are specialized to regulate motor control or emotional responses, to hold information in long-term or short-term (working) memory, and so on. But complex behaviors, such as the way that a monkey protects his eyes from intruding objects, are regulated by neural networks formed by circuits linking populations of neurons in neuroanatomical structures that may be distributed throughout the brain (Mesulam, 1990). Observable complex behaviors, such as looking at and reaching for an object, are regulated by neural circuits that constitute distributed networks linking activity in many different neuroanatomical structures. As Mesulam notes, "complex behavior is mapped at the level of multifocal neural systems rather than specific anatomical sites, giving rise to brain-behavior relationships that are both localized and distributed" (1990, p. 598). Therefore, it is impossible to localize the "seat" of a complex behavior. A particular neuroanatomical structure can support different neuronal populations that project to neurons in different parts of the brain, thereby supporting circuits that regulate different aspects of behavior.

In other words, although specific operations may be performed in particular parts of the brain, these operations must be integrated into a *network* that regulates an observable aspect of behavior. And so, a particular aspect of behavior usually involves activity in neuroanatomical structures distributed throughout the brain.

Converging evidence from studies that relate brain activity to behavior in many species shows that there is a class of "functional neural systems" that generate appropriate, timely responses to environmental challenges and opportunities. These distributed neural systems monitor incoming sensory information and modify or generate goal-directed motor activity. The postulated human FLS is a particular example of this class of functional neural systems. For example, as we shall see, it is a distributed network that includes basal ganglia neuroanatomical structures that play a part in regulating sequencing when people move their fingers (Cunnington et al., 1995), talk (Lieberman et al., 1992), attempt to comprehend distinctions in meaning conveyed by syntax (Lieberman, Friedman, and Feldman, 1990; Lieberman et al., 1992; Grossman et al., 1991, 1993; Natsopoulos et al., 1993), and solve cognitive problems (Lange et al., 1992; Mentzel et al., 1998; Pickett et al., 1998). The basal ganglia structures that perform the same basic operation, sequencing, in these different aspects of behavior support segregated neuronal populations that project to segregated neuronal populations in other subcortical structures and cortical areas (Alexander, DeLong, and Strick, 1986; Parent, 1986; Cummings, 1993; Middleton and Strick, 1994; Graybiel et al., 1994; Marsden and Obeso, 1994; Wise, 1997). Since natural selection selects for timely responses to environmental challenges (otherwise you may be eaten), functional neural systems channel sensory information directly to neuronal populations that mediate appropriate, timely motor responses to stimuli. Therefore, it is not surprising to find that the FLS also provides direct access to the primary information—auditory, visual, pragmatic, and motoric—coded in a word (Just and Carpenter, 1992; MacDonald, 1994; Martin et al., 1995).

Moreover, studies of the neural activity implicated in motor control show that circuits are formed as an animal or human "learns" to execute a task (e.g., Sanes and Donoghue, 1994, 1996, 1997; Karni et al., 1995, 1998; Pascual-Leone et al., 1995; Sanes et al., 1995; Nudo et al., 1996; Classen et al., 1998). The studies that will be discussed suggest that the circuits of the FLS that specify the specific sounds, words, and syntax of language are learned as children and adults are exposed to a particular language or languages. The process would be similar to that by which a person learns to play a violin or a dog to retrieve balls. Although "sensitive" or "critical" periods exist within which a skill such as speaking English can be readily acquired, similar sensitive periods limit the acquisition of binocular vision or learning to play the violin skillfully. Other sensitive or "critical" periods exist in which children can acquire language after massive damage destroys parts of the brain that usually form part of the FLS. Current neurobehavioral data demonstrate both the plastic and activity-dependent nature of the specific knowledge represented in cortical structures and the possibility that alternate neuroantomical structures are enlisted for language after brain damage. These biological facts all argue against neural structures that code innate linguistic knowledge such as the hypothetical "Universal Grammar" proposed by Noam Chomsky (1972, 1986).

In other words, my claim is that the neuroanatomical substrate of the FLS is part of the human genotype; the particular neural circuits that code words, regulate syntax, control speech production, and perceive speech sounds are shaped in the course of development in particular linguistic environments. In brief, the neural architecture of the human FLS involves *neuroanatomical structures,* various areas of the cortex and subcortical structures that have been discerned using traditional anatomical procedures, and *neuronal circuits* that can be mapped by means of tracer and electrophysiologic techniques at a microscopic level. Particular neuroanatomical structures appear to perform specific computations, but a given neuroanatomical structure can support many different circuits that project to different assemblages of neuroanatomical structures. Circuits regulate particular aspects of linguistic behavior, but the architecture of a given neural circuit that regulates a particular aspect of behavior is not necessarily either logical or parsimonious. As Mayr (1982) notes, the logic of biology inherently reflects the opportunistic nature of biological evolution. Neuroanatomical structures that were adapted to carry out one function were modified to regulate new behaviors that contributed to biological fitness, the survival of progeny. Thus the model proposed here has the following features:

1. Human language is regulated by a neural functional language system (FLS), similar in principle to the functional systems that regulate other aspects of behavior in human beings and other animals. It is a distributed rather than a strictly hierarchical system; similar operations are performed in parallel, redundantly, in different anatomical sites. The system is dynamic, enlisting additional resources as task complexity increases.
2. Speech is central to human language. The FLS regulates both the motor commands that underlie speech and the perception of speech, bringing a listener's "knowledge" of the articulatory constraints of speech production to bear on the interpretation of the acoustic signal. The FLS accesses words from the brain's dictionary through their sound pattern (or manual signs for these alternate phonetic systems) and maintains words in verbal working memory by means of a rehearsal mechanism (silent speech) in which words are internally modeled by the neural mechanisms that regulate the production of speech or manual signs.

3. The mark of evolution on the FLS is apparent. Subcortical basal ganglia structures usually associated with motor control are key elements of the FLS, reflecting its probable evolutionary history. Natural selection operated on motor control systems that provided timely responses to environmental challenges and opportunities in ancestral hominid species. These subcortical structures continue to play a part in regulating aspects of human behavior such as bipedal locomotion and manual motor control. Their continued involvement in different aspects of behavior again reflects the mechanism of evolution noted by Charles Darwin in 1859—organs adapted to a particular function or functions take on new tasks. Other neuroanatomical structures of the FLS play a part in aspects of human cognition outside the domain of language. Therefore, natural selection that enhanced the computational power of a neuroanatomical structure that plays a part in regulating different aspects of behavior may enhance its role in all of these behaviors. Thus, enhanced linguistic ability cannot be totally differentiated from enhanced cognitive ability and motor activity.
4. Finally, many aspects of human language are not unique attributes of present-day humans, anatomically modern *Homo sapiens*. Lexical and syntactic abilities exist to a degree in present-day apes. Archaic hominids such as *Erectus*-grade hominids and the Neanderthals must have possessed vocal language; otherwise there would have been no basis for adaptations that enhanced the efficiency and saliency of speech production in anatomically modern *Homo sapiens*.

Modularity and the Functional Neural System

The neural architecture of the functional language system differs profoundly from that implied by current "modular" theories of mind (Chomsky, 1980a, 1980b, 1986; Fodor, 1983). First it is essential to note the subtle but crucial difference between the meaning of the word *module* as it is used in neurobiological studies and those that attempt to reconcile experimental data with Chomskian linguistic theory, such as Levelt (1989), Jackendoff (1994), and Pinker (1994). Current modular views of the neural bases of language derive from Paul Broca (1861), who claimed that he had found the "seat" of language in a particular part of the neocortex. Broca's claim was retained by Chomsky (1980a, 1980b), who stated that the human brain contains a unique localized "language organ," which regulates language independently of the neural mechanisms that are implicated in other aspects of human behavior or the behavior of other animals. Indeed, in this respect Chomsky owes much to Descartes, who in his letter of 1646 to the Marquis of Newcastle stated that "language belongs to man alone." Chomsky focused on language "competence" or "knowledge of language" rather than the processes by which people make use of their knowledge of language.

Fodor's (1983) modular theory, which derives from Chomsky's model, attempts to account for the *processes* that might be involved in communicating or thinking by means of language. Fodor's modular theory reduces to a set of "black boxes," each of which carries out a process such as speech perception or stores a knowledge base such as the rules of syntax. Each hypothetical module has an independent status. The modules are "black boxes" since Fodor makes no claims concerning the neural machinery in each module. Fodor's modules do not differ in principle from the "faculties" of the brain that nineteenth-century phrenologists mapped onto skulls (Spurzheim, 1815). Phrenologists partitioned the exterior of the brain into discrete areas. Each area bore the label of the particular aspect of behavior, veneration, anger, honesty, and so forth, that it supposedly regulated. The primary difference between phrenological maps and current modular maps is that the labels are different and refer to areas of the neocortex. In modular, neophrenological linguistic theory, various cortical areas are the "seats" of syntax, phonology, the lexicon, and so forth. All aspects of observed behavior ultimately are localized.

The studies that will be discussed in this book show that this view does not correctly characterize the brain. It is apparent that various parts of the human brain carry out particular operations. For example, some areas of the cortex support local circuits that code the shape of an object, other areas code its color, while other areas code its position. However, these operations do not necessarily correspond to our intuitions concerning the physical senses: intuitively vision is holistic. We see objects as entities that have a shape and color in specific locations. Our intuitions concerning behavior and thought, for which we have words such as vision, hearing, speech, and language, date back at least to the time of the Greek philosophers of the classical period who formulated theories concerning the nature of the physical universe and the human mind. Although many of their theories have been supplanted, their views concerning the mind-brain persist in present-day linguistic "modular" views of relationships between brain, mind, and language (Chomsky, 1980a, 1980b, 1986; Fodor, 1983). Linguists often assume that their intuitions concerning the various components that together constitute human language directly map onto various discrete parts of the brain that independently regulate phonetics, phonology, syntax, semantics, the lexicon, and so on. But intuition, though it may reflect a long scholarly tradition, is a poor data base for any scientific theory.

According to Fodor (1983), the processing modules of the mind are "encapsulated." The term "encapsulation," like other aspects of Fodor's theory, seems to be borrowed from the design principles of military electronic devices and the digital computers that were developed during and shortly after World War II. Early military radars were difficult to maintain because there was no invariant, one-to-one relationship between a discrete circuit element and a "behavioral attribute" of the radar. Vacuum tubes were prone to failure, so designers kept the total number of tubes to a minimum by designing "switches" that could place a given vacuum tube into different circuits. The same vacuum tube, for example, might form part of several circuits. In one circuit its failure could disrupt the radar's ability to spot aircraft at a distance. The same failure in another circuit would make it impossible to accurately direct gunfire at a nearby target. It was necessary to understand the details of the radar's circuit design to make timely repairs. Modular design was introduced to allow quick, easy repair. Military radars were designed with modular, plug-in circuit boards. Each modular board contained the circuits and vacuum tubes that carried out a specific operation such as the circuits that calculated the velocity of a target aircraft and the circuits that displayed information on the cathode-ray tube. Technicians could repair a malfunctioning radar set by observing the nature of the malfunction—for example, a defective display—and simply replacing one circuit board. Modular design principles were carried over into computer systems. If a computer's printer interface isn't working, the printer module can be exchanged, additional memory plugged in, newer computational chips substituted for older versions. Encapsulated electronic circuit boards also were introduced during World War II to protect electronic components from tropical humidity, dirt, water, and so on. Electronic circuit boards were literally placed in capsules of epoxy resin, which limited access to their electronic components and operations.

The concept of encapsulation is a central feature of Fodor's modular theory; it is impossible to influence the operations within each hypothetical module. Encapsulation may characterize certain neural circuits, for example those that monitor oxygen levels in the bloodstream and cerebrospinal fluid (Bouhuys, 1974), but it isn't necessarily a general condition. As we shall see, one of the properties of subcortical basal ganglia is that they interrupt ongoing activity in a circuit in response to new information. The process occurs in basal ganglia structures that regulate manual motor control, speech production, the comprehension of distinctions in meaning conveyed by syntax, and other aspects of cognition.

The hypothetical modules of current psycholinguistic theories, furthermore, have "shallow outputs"—the input information available to a module is not preserved in the module's output. For example, according to modular theories the comprehension of language involves the chained activity of a sequence of encapsulated modules; speech is first processed by a "speech-to-phonetic" module in which the incoming acoustic signal is transformed into a phonetic representation. The phonetic representation, in turn, is the input to a lexical module, which has no access to the primary acoustic information that was available to the phonetic module, and so on. But recent studies of lexical access in human subjects show that this is not the case. The data of Andruski, Blumstein, and Burton (1994), for example, show that lexical access is in fact affected by "subphonetic" acoustic information, supposedly isolated in the hypothetical "speech-to-phonetic" module.

Again, according to current modular theory, the "linguistic" modules involved in speech perception have nothing to do with other "auditory" modules. Indeed, since other animals do not talk, some modular theorists appear to assume that auditory processes have nothing to do with language processing. Liberman and Mattingly (1985), for example, propose a hypothetical "speech perception" module that carries out operations specific to human speech. Other hypothetical "auditory" modules would carry out computations relating to auditory processes such as locating the direction of a sound made by a footstep. However, it is clear that the auditory process that humans and many other mammals use to localize the source of a sound (Hirsch and Sherrick, 1961) also structures the linguistic decision by which we differentiate the word *bat* from *pat*. Kuhl (1981) has shown that chinchillas, monkeys, and human infants, children, and adults partition the acoustic signals that convey this distinction in much the same manner because they all make use of a basic constraint of the mammalian auditory system.

Moreover, the feed-forward and -back connections observed in all cortical areas (e.g., Bear, Conners, and Paradiso, 1996; Paus et al., 1996) provide direct anatomical evidence against the sequential operations presupposed in modular processing models. It also is evident that the "computations" or operations carried out in particular neuroanatomical structures have distributed representations, particularly in the cortex, where almost no lesion completely destroys a function, only degrading performance (Elman et al., 1996). Biological brains simply do not conform to the design principles of radar sets or conventional digital computers.

Linguistic Theory

Several aspects of current linguistic practice will be discussed in the following chapters.

Universal Grammar and Syntax

Syntax is to Chomsky and most linguists the feature of human language that makes it unique. The central claim of the Chomskian school is that human syntactic ability derives from a specialized, genetically transmitted syntax module or "organ" of the human brain (Chomsky, 1986). It instantiates the "Universal Grammar," a set of innate "principles and parameters" that exist in all human brains. The Universal Grammar specifies the total range of morphologic and syntactic rules that can occur in any given human language. Children supposedly do not learn the rules that govern syntax by means of general cognitive processes such as imitation or associative learning. The principles and parameters coded in the hypothetical Universal Grammar are instead triggered to yield the correct grammar of a particular language as a child is exposed to normal discourse (Chomsky, 1986; Jackendoff, 1994; Pinker, 1994).

As we shall see, it is difficult to reconcile a Universal Grammar instantiated in genetically specified neural structures with studies that show that children acquire language after suffering brain damage which destroys the neuroanatomical structures that usually regulate language. Other structures take on the task through a general process of neural plasticity (Elman et al., 1996; Bates et al., 1997; Bates, Vicari, and Trauner, 1999). Neural linguistic plasticity is not limited to children. Similar neural plasticity resulted in a sixty-year-old male's retaining language after the total destruction of Wernicke's area (Lieberman et al., in submission). Still, clinical studies consistently note that aphasic victims of strokes that destroy cortical areas, producing transient loss of language, often recover (Stuss and Benson, 1986).

Algorithmic Solutions

Universal Grammar is not necessary to account for human linguistic ability, nor is it a necessary component of formal linguistic theory. However, it has become linked to formal linguistic theory through the deficiencies of its algorithmic methodology. Chomsky's (1957) initial goal was to describe the grammatical "rules" or "transformations" that mediated between a hypothetical "deep," semantic level at which the meaning of a sentence is represented in the human mind, and a "surface" level that described spoken, grammatical sentences. The transformations were stated as formal, mathematical algorithms that mediated between the two levels. The "kernel" sentence *Susan saw the boy,* close to the deep semantic level, could be transformed into the surface-level passive sentence *The boy was seen by Susan* by means of an algorithm, a "passive transformational rule."

Most aspects of Chomsky's 1957 theory have been modified, but all subsequent versions of generative grammar have retained the proposition that a set of algorithms, instantiated in the human brain, will generate the "grammatical" sentences of a particular language or dialect, rejecting ungrammatical sentences. Many important insights concerning the nature of language have since been discovered. However, despite forty years of effort, linguists have failed to discover any set of algorithms, rules of grammar, that suffice to describe the grammatical sentences and rule out the ungrammatical sentences of any natural language. Although English is the language that has been most intensively studied by linguists, the set of English sentences that can be described by formal grammatical "rules" has not significantly changed in forty years. As Ray Jackendoff, one of Chomsky's advocates, notes: "Thousands of linguists throughout the world have been trying for decades to figure out the principles behind the grammatical patterns of various languages . . . But any linguist will tell you that we are nowhere near a complete account of the mental grammar for any language" (1994, p. 26). Paradoxically, the *failure* of linguists to discover a set of algorithms that can specify the grammatical sentences of any human language is taken as evidence for the existence of an innate Universal Grammar. The logic of this argument, which Jakendoff (1994) repeats, is that whereas young children can acquire the rules of grammar of any human language without any formal instruction, highly trained linguists cannot describe these rules after decades of study. It supposedly follows that the failed scholarly endeavor demonstrates that the rules of grammar *must* be part of human innate knowledge. How else could a child acquire language, when so many learned scholars fail to discern the rules that regulate language? With equal logic we could argue that the failure of engineers to devise computer-guided machines that can attach bumpers to slightly misaligned cars on an assembly line with the facility of human workers, shows that the human brain must have an innate "bumper-installation-instruction-set" organ. The answer that seems more likely, in light of current neurobiological data, is that biological brains do not carry out algorithmic processes. The chapters that follow will discuss this issue.

But the general consensus among formal linguists is that language, especially syntax, is not learned by children. The principles governing the acquisition of syntax are supposedly part of the innate Universal Grammar, coded by our genes. The linguistic environment that a child is exposed to supposedly acts to "trigger" or "release" knowledge of language that is already coded at birth in every human brain (Chomsky, 1986). But claiming an innate basis for syntax does not really solve the problem. One must then account for the properties of the hypothetical innate Universal Grammar. Therefore, the focus of many linguistic and developmental studies (such as Pinker, 1984) has been redirected toward discovering the properties of the Universal Grammar. It is difficult to see how one could discover the properties of a Universal Grammar without first being able to describe the syntax of all human languages. If the full range of grammatical sentences that occur in different languages cannot be described, then how can linguists be certain that they have discovered "universal properties"?

Competence, Performance, and Theories of Data

Yet another deficiency of current linguistic theory is that it incorporates features that make it impossible to test theory against data. As the philosopher of science Mario Bunge (1984, 1985) noted, linguistic theories commonly are tested against *theories* of data rather than against actual data. This aspect of linguistic practice is not limited to Chomsky and his adherents. In the early decades of the present century the Swiss linguist Saussure (1959) started the study of language down a slippery slope when he declared that the true objective of linguistic research was to understand phenomena that reflected *la langue,* knowledge of language. Other linguistic data supposedly reflected extraneous events, *parole,* that could safely be ignored. External, objective principles that would differentiate langue from *parole* were never specified. The *langue/parole* distinction, governing the relationship between data and linguistic theory, was elaborated in the Chomskian era. Certain data supposedly reflect linguistic "competence," knowledge of language, while other data reflect "performance" effects that can be ignored (Chomsky, 1986). The *langue/parole*–competence/performance distinction is necessary because sentences conforming to the "rules" of grammar proposed by linguists generally are not produced when people converse. Indeed, transcripts of lectures delivered by distinguished scholars reveal departures from the grammatically "correct" sentences that form the data base for linguistic theories. Grammatical knowledge of language supposedly may be attained by means of intuitive introspection. But one person's intuition is not necessarily another's. And in practice, as Bunge notes, the competence/performance distinction is often used to reject data that falsify the current theory. In the course of time, as generative theory has changed, "crucial" data that formerly demonstrated the "psychological reality" of the theory became irrelevant "performance" effects.

For example, psycholinguistic studies such as Miller (1963) and Savin and Perchonock (1965) were cited by Chomsky and his supporters as crucial evidence for the psychological reality of "Generative Grammars" based on Chomsky's 1957 theory. These experimental studies showed that English-speaking subjects took more time to comprehend or recall a passive sentence such as *Susan was seen by John,* which according to Chomsky's 1957 "Generative Grammar" theory had been "generated" from the kernel sentence *John saw Susan* through application of the passive "transformational rule." According to contemporary Chomskian theory, the meaning of a sentence was represented in the underlying kernel sentence. Therefore, the increased time that a listener needed to comprehend a passive sentence apparently reflected the mental processes involved in undoing the passive transformation to arrive at the kernel sentence. However, these "crucial" data abruptly became irrelevant "performance" effects when Chomsky's 1972 linguistic theory dispensed with kernel sentences.

A further refinement of this exclusionary principle is the distinction between "core" and "peripheral" grammar. In practice, the core grammar is the fragment of the linguistic corpus that conforms to the algorithms proposed by a particular linguistic theory. The "peripheral" grammar is the body of linguistic data that the theory cannot account for. William Croft

(1991), for example, documents the fragmentary data bases and arbitrary criteria on which formalist Chomskian grammarians base the supposed "universal constraints" of grammar. As Croft notes, "certain constructions are separated out as the ones that manifest the universal distinctions and the others are treated as 'superficial'" (1991, p. 24).

Apart from its arbitrary nature, the competence-performance distinction is biologically implausible. Unless we adopt a creationist position we must acknowledge that the neural bases of human language evolved by means of the evolutionary mechanisms that Charles Darwin proposed in 1859.[1] Although some biologists (e.g., Gould and Eldridge, 1977) have placed more emphasis on the pace of evolution, Darwin's theories are still the keystone of biology (Mayr, 1982). Recent studies confirm the central role of Darwinian natural selection in evolution. Natural selection operates quickly, favoring variations that, for example, changed the shape and feeding habits of stickleback fish when a new competitor forced the species to adapt to a different ecological niche (Schluter, 1994). Therefore, linguists and cognitive scientists who wish to account for a Universal Grammar have proposed that it was shaped by natural selection (Pinker and Bloom, 1990; Pinker, 1994). However, as Darwin stressed, natural selection acts on overt behavior that increases biological "fitness," the survival of more progeny of particular individuals, not on unexpressed competence for some behavior. Therefore, performance effects that describe actual linguistic behavior cannot be ignored if Universal Grammar evolved by means of natural selection, as Pinker and Bloom (1990), Pinker (1994), and Williams and Wakefield (1995) have proposed.[2]

Objectives

This book will not attempt to explain how the brain or mind works. We simply do not know how biological brains work. However, we can reject some theories. The studies reviewed in the following chapters show that the traditional model of the brain bases of language, Geschwind's (1970) reformulation of Lichtheim's (1885) theory, is at best incomplete. These explicate some aspects of the FLS and, by revealing gaps in our current knowledge, suggest further studies.

Many of the cortical neuroanatomical structures that sustain the neural circuits regulating language have been identified (e.g., Geschwind, 1970; Stuss and Benson, 1986; Caplan, 1987; Fuster, 1989; Grafman, 1989; Carramaza and Hillis, 1990; Mesulam, 1990; Damasio, 1991; Blumstein, 1994,

1995; Awh et al., 1996). I will focus on other recent data, complementing these findings, which indicate that subcortical basal ganglia structures play a central role in the FLS. A central objective will be to fill in the "striatum" box, modifying the flow lines that diagram the exchange of information in Mesulam's (1990) network model of the possible neural bases of language. (See Figure I-1.) The primary flow of information and neural processing appears to involve circuits through, rather than parallel to, basal ganglia structures.

But we are only at the threshold of understanding how the human brain works. The techniques that would allow us to map out the circuits that regulate human language do not yet exist. Neural circuits can be mapped only for aspects of behavior that occur in animals that lack spoken language. Therefore, a complete specification of the neural circuits or neuroanatomical structures that constitute the FLS cannot be provided. What is offered here is a starting point, a theory that relates phenomena that are seemingly unrelated, such as why the pattern of deficits associated with the syndrome of Broca's aphasia involves certain aspects of speech production, lexical access,

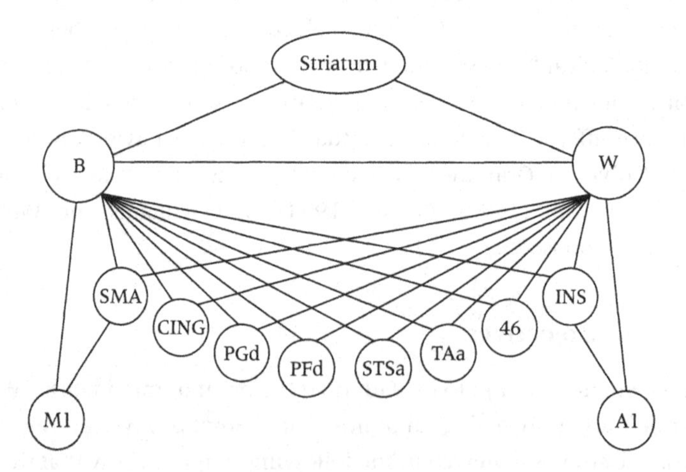

Figure I-1. Mesulam's network model of the neural bases of language. The circled symbols represent cortical areas or neuroanatomical structures; the lines represent the information flow. B = Broca's area, W = Wernicke's area, M1 and A1 = primary motor and auditory cortex, SMA = supplementary motor area, CING = cingulate gyrus, PGd and PFd = dorsal and ventral parts of cortical areas PG and PF, STSa = anterior bank of superior temporal sulcus, TAa = anterior part of superior temporal gyrus auditory association area, 46 = Brodmann's area 46, INS = insula. The striatum includes the basal ganglia. (After Mesulam, 1990.)

and the comprehension of distinctions in meaning conveyed by syntax, why similar effects occur in Parkinson's disease, why children are able to learn language after massive cortical damage, why recovery from certain types of brain damage is problematic, and why aged people who speak slowly also have difficulty comprehending distinctions in meaning conveyed by complex syntax or long sentences.

I will also attempt to convince readers that it is worth considering the evolution of the brain if we wish to understand the neural basis of human language. Charles Darwin in *On the Origin of Species* did more than to introduce the concept of evolution. As Ernst Mayr (1982) noted, Darwin developed the science of evolutionary biology. We clearly lack any direct knowledge of the behavior of the extinct hominids who lived 5 million years ago. However, we can follow in Darwin's footsteps, studying the behavior, morphology, and physiology of species that have some of the "primitive" features that occur in them and us. For example, no one would dispute the fact that we can learn much concerning hand-eye motor coordination by studying the neural mechanisms that regulate this activity in monkeys. Although the brains of human beings differ from those of monkeys, there are common, primitive features that reflect our common ancestry. There obviously are "derived" features that differentiate the brains of human beings from monkeys, but we can determine some aspects of human behavior that derive from these primitive characteristics. Thus, in the light of evolution it is not surprising to find that neuroanatomical structures traditionally associated with motor control in humans are essential components of the FLS. They reflect the continuity of evolution; the neural substrate that confers human cognitive ability appears to derive from the systems that produce appropriate, timely motor responses in response to changing environmental challenges and opportunities.

Current neurobiological studies have provided new insights into the brain bases of human language and cognitive ability. The shared insights of neurobiology, cognitive science, linguistics, and evolutionary biology can lead us to a better understanding of the biological bases and nature of human language and thought. Darwin took care in 1859 to point out the "imperfections" of his theory. Imperfections certainly must exist in the functional language system theory presented here. But the FLS theory can furnish a starting point for a better approximation of the neural bases of human language.

The most desirable outcome would be a new era of biological linguistics, one involving cooperative research among linguists, cognitive scientists, and neurobiologists. Instead of relying on intuitions of grammaticality, linguists could determine how and what people actually communicate. Then concerned cognitive scientists and neurobiologists could determine whether biologically plausible models of the human brain can account for linguistic data that capture the full capacity of human language and thought.

CHAPTER 1

Functional Neural Systems

Ernst Mayr, in his superb preface to the 1964 facsimile edition of *On the Origin of Species,* points out that Darwin introduced the paradigm governing modern research. Theories are based on preliminary data, are tested against additional data, and, if they are useful, lead to refined theories that explain a greater range of phenomena. Data and theory are inextricably linked. A theory is necessarily formulated on the basis of initial data. Therefore, all theories are inherently structured by the technical constraints that limit experiment and observation. A theory is then subject to test by further experiment and observation, but the theory's explicit and implicit assumptions inherently determine the experiments and techniques that appear to be relevant. Subsequent data usually result in modification of the theory. The process is neither strictly deductive or inductive. Experimental data do not merely serve to refute or confirm the predictions of a theory. Experimental techniques, the interpretation of data, and the theoretical claims deriving from these data are constrained by a common set of implicit and explicit assumptions.

This chapter surveys the historical background and experimental techniques that pertain both to traditional, neophrenological theories and to the theory proposed here to explain the nature and evolution of the brain bases of language. It also briefly reviews the basic anatomy of the human brain, neuronal theory, distributed neural networks, and functional neural systems. Various parts of the discussion are, of course, unnecessary for particular specialists, who may find similar background discussions concerning other topics helpful.

Background

Finding Your Way around the Brain

Like other aspects of human morphology and physiology, the design of the human brain is not logical or optimal. Although language is one of the most recent "derived" features of *Homo sapiens,* it is becoming apparent that phylogenetically "primitive" neuroanatomical structures found in the brains of "lower" animals, such as the cerebellum and basal ganglia, play a part in regulating human language and thought. Converging evidence from many independent studies shows that the basal ganglia, which are buried deep within the cerebrum, clearly play a part in human language and thought. These primitive structures, which derive from the brains of amphibians and reptiles (Parent, 1986; Marin, Smeets, and Gonzalez, 1998), appear to have been modified in the course of evolution for these ends and to work in concert with various regions of the neocortex and cortex.

Much of the brain is divided into two roughly equal halves, "cerebral hemispheres" along the front (anterior) to back (posterior) axis. And virtually all the brain's neuroanatomical structures come in pairs, one in each side. In quadripedal animals, the term "rostral" also refers to the front of the brain (literally toward the "beak" in Latin), while "caudal" refers to the back (Latin for "tail"). The direction toward the back is "dorsal" (the Latin word for "back"), while the direction toward the stomach is "ventral." Structures closer to the midline of the brain are "medial"; those farther out from the midline are "lateral." The internal structure is generally viewed in "sections" that can be obtained either by slicing the brain or by the computerized imaging techniques (CT and MRI scans) reviewed below. The section that is formed by splitting the brain in two along the anterior-posterior midline is the "sagittal" plane. Sections parallel to the midsagittal plane are "parasagittal." Sections parallel to the ground are "horizontal." Sections perpendicular to the midsagital and horizontal planes are "coronal" or "frontal."

The neocortex, the outer layer of the cerebrum, consists of right and left hemispheres. The part of the cortex lying under the forehead is the frontal lobe. The sylvian fissure, a deep groove, separates the frontal region from the temporal lobe, while the shallower central sulcus marks the border between the frontal and parietal lobes. The neocortex, which occurs only in mammals, has a characteristic structure of neurons arranged in six layers. (See Figure 1–1.) The "paleocortex" is located within the posterior part of the frontal lobe. Basal ganglia structures, which are located within the cerebrum, are also represented right and left. Basal ganglia derive from structures found in reptiles and amphibians, but in mammals they are more differentiated, larger, and support neuronal circuits that connect to cortical areas. Basal ganglia participate in motor control, the regulation of affect, language, and cognition. The thalamus, hippocampus, cerebellum, and other subcortical structures also connect to different cortical areas and subcortical structures. Pathways channeling sensory information up to the brain and signals down to midbrain structures project from many of these neuroanatomical structures. Pathways to the spinal cord also project from certain neocortical areas. Electrical stimulation of motor cortex, for example, elicits the contraction of muscles via direct pathways from this cortical area to the spinal cord.

Neurons

The elementary computing elements that make up the nervous systems of animals are neurons. The basic structure of each neuron consists of a cell

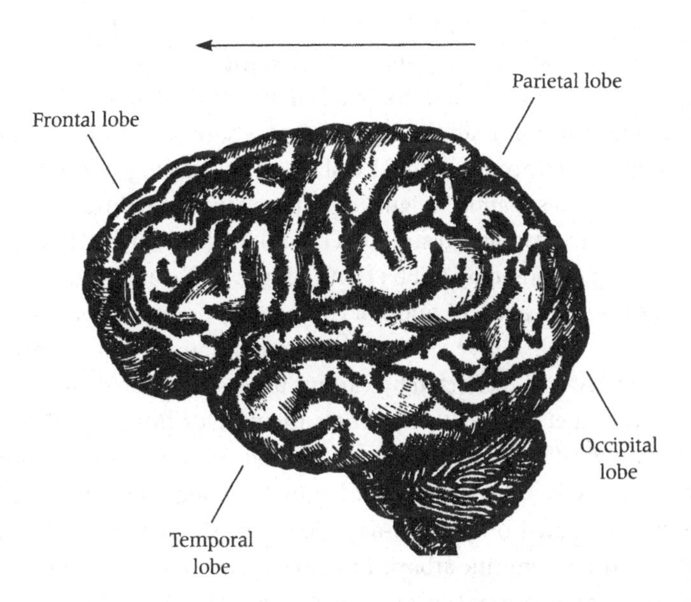

Figure 1-1. Lateral view of the left hemisphere of the human brain, showing the major regions of the neocortex. The arrow points to the anterior, frontal regions.

body, or soma (the two terms are used interchangeably—a common occurrence in anatomical terminology). Neurons interconnect by means of dendrites and axons. A cluster of dendrites (the Greek terminology refers to the treelike image formed by the dendrites that branch out from each cell body) is associated with each neuron. A cortical neuron typically receives inputs on these dendrites from a few thousand other neurons. Each neuron has an output axon, which again typically is arborized and transmits information to a few thousand neurons. Incoming axons from other neurons transmit information into the dendritic tree of a neuron through chemical synapses on the dendritic tree and the cell body. The traditional view of the dendrites was that they were biological analogues of electrical wires that simply transmitted information without modifying it. However, it is becoming evident that dendrites play a role in modifying synaptic weights. Synapses are the structures that determine the degree to which an incoming signal will cause the cell body to generate an electrical pulse, the action potential or "spike" that it transmits out without decrement on its axon. The output action potential can be visualized as an abruptly rising electrical spike when it's monitored by microelectrodes, exceedingly fine electrodes that usually are positioned in or near a neuron.

Both inhibitory and excitory synapses exist. They respectively result in an incoming signal's having less or more effect in triggering an action potential. A loose analogy would be to think of a synapse as the biological equivalent of the volume control of an audio amplifier whose setting determines the extent to which an incoming signal will result in its being transformed into output sound. The synaptic weights of a population of neurons may, in effect, constitute an adaptable distributed memory. The neuronal basis of associative learning proposed by Hebb (1949) hinges on the modification of synaptic weights by the axon of one cell consistently and repeatedly firing the axon of another cell. However, long-term potentiation, that is, changes in synaptic weights, is also effected by various processes in the dendrites themselves (Markram et al., 1997). Dendrites themselves (Magee and Johnson, 1997) are implicated in the process of Hebbian synaptic modification that appears to be the key to associative learning in biological brains, and that is imperfectly simulated on present-day computer simulations of neural net activity. Extensive dendritic arborization exists everywhere, connecting various neuronal populations, possibly linking circuits.[1] Massive interconnections link most cortical areas with considerable, though not complete, reciprocity (Bear, Conners, and Paradiso, 1996).

Mind-Brain Theories

The traditional view of the neural bases of complex behaviors derives from phrenology. Phrenologists claimed that different parts of the cranium were the "seats" of various aspects of behavior or character (Gall, 1809; Spurzheim, 1815). Although phrenology is usually dismissed as a quack science, basic phrenological concepts persist. Neophrenological theories do not claim that a bump on a person's skull can tell you that he is honest. However, they claim that activity confined to a particular part of the brain regulates a complex aspect of behavior. The best-known neophrenological theory arguably is the Broca-Wernicke model of the brain bases of human language.[2]

If one assumes that discrete localized regions of the brain *in themselves* regulate an observable aspect of behavior, it follows that removing or destroying that region should disrupt the behavior. Paul Broca (1861) studied a patient, "Tan," who had suffered a series of strokes that caused extensive brain damage including but not limited to one part of the brain, "the third frontal convolution," an anterior area of the neocortex. However, Broca concluded that damage to this area (Broca's area) was the basis of the patient's language deficits. Tan's most obvious linguistic problem was his limited speech ability; the only utterance that he was able to produce was the syllable *tan*. Broca and his successors, Wernicke (1874) and Lichtheim (1885), essentially translated the phrenological theories of Gall (1809) and Spurzheim (1815) to cortical areas. According to the Broca-Wernicke model proposed by Lichtheim (1885), spoken language is perceived in Wernicke's area, a posterior temporal region associated with auditory perception. Information is then transmitted via a cortical pathway to Broca's region, adjacent to cortical areas implicated in motor control. Broca's region is the hypothetical neural site regulating speech production. Geschwind's (1970) theory, which continues to shape brain and language theories, is essentially a restatement of Lichtheim's views.

Perhaps the most compelling reason for the persistence of this and other phrenological theories is the force of analogy. Historically, the most complex piece of machinery of an epoch serves as a metaphor for the brain. The metaphor seems to take on a life of its own and becomes a neurophysiological model. In the eighteenth and nineteenth centuries the brain was often compared to a clock or chronometer. During the first part of the twentieth century the model usually was a telephone exchange, and since the 1950s a digital computer. Mechanical-biological analogies, of course, are not limited to neurophysiology. Physicians bled feverish patients in the early nineteenth century because of a false analogy between blood temperature and steam engines. Early steam engines frequently exploded as pressure increased at high operating temperatures. Safety valves then were invented that released superheated pressure. Hence it followed that bleeding would reduce temperature. As a result of this false analogy, the chances of survival for soldiers wounded at Waterloo were greater if they had not been treated by surgeons immediately after the battle. In its own way, the analogy between biological brains and digital computers is as fatal for understanding the neural bases of human language.

The discrete, localized, modular structural architecture of computers is reflected in current modular mind-brain theories of language. The central processing unit of a digital computer is a discrete device, RAM memory is discrete, and hard drives are discrete, "modular" devices. These discrete devices translate to discrete areas of the neocortex and other parts of the brain. The serial, algorithmic, computational architecture of the digital computer likewise translates into modular linguistic and psycholinguistic theories. Modular models claim that language is comprehended and produced by means of a series of independent operations. The first stage in the comprehension of spoken language hypothetically is a process whereby phonetic units or "features" (Jakobson et al., 1952) are derived from the acoustic signal, perhaps mediated by vocal tract modeling (Liberman et al., 1967). High-level "top-down" information (the semantic and pragmatic constraints conveyed by the words or word fragments that are being specified by incoming acoustic information) supposedly provides only secondary corrective information. However, experimental data show that these claims are incorrect. Human speech, including that of university professors, generally is a sloppy, underspecified signal that deviates from textbook phonetic transcriptions. Tape-recorded lectures are notoriously difficult to transcribe because speakers almost always underspecify the acoustic cues that convey phonetic contrasts. Even "well-formed" speech recorded under ideal conditions is often completely incomprehensible until a listener hears at least a 600-millisecond segment (Pollack and Pickett, 1963). Yet we are generally unaware of these problems because we "fill in" missing information, overriding acoustic phenomena that conflict with our internally generated hypotheses concerning what was *probably* said, and the probability involves a weighting of semantic and pragmatic information derived from parallel, highly redundant processing. Many of these phenomena can be explained if we take into account the distributed, parallel processing that appears to typify biological brains.

Distributed Neural Networks

Starting in the late 1950s various efforts were made to model parallel processing using "computing machinery" that attempted to capture some aspects of the neurophysiology of biological brains. These models ultimately derive from Hebb's (1949) theory of synaptic modification. Hebb proposed that the activity of neurons tends to become correlated when they continually respond to some stimuli that share common properties. Hebb suggested that when "cell A is near enough to excite a cell B and repeatedly or persistently takes part in firing it, some growth or metabolic change takes place in one or both cells such that A's efficiency as one of the cells firing B is increased" (1949, p. 62).

Hebb's theory is consistent with experimental data showing that conduction across the synapse is enhanced as animals are exposed to paired stimuli. This process has been experimentally verified in both complex (Bear, Cooper, and Ebner, 1987) and phylogenetically primitive animals. Mollusks can be trained using a Pavlovian technique in which an electric shock is paired with a hitherto benign stimulus. Synaptic modification is apparent in *Aplysia californicus* exposed to "smells" or "tastes" (essence of squid) followed by electric shocks. The trained mollusks "learn" to run away and squirt clouds of ink (Carew, Walters, and Kandel, 1981).

Figure 1-2 shows a simple multilayered neural network.[3] The individual input units are triggered by particular inputs and "fire," thereby transmitting signals to the hidden units through modifiable connections. The "connection weights" between the units model the modifiable synaptic connections that exist in a biological brain. The connection weights are modified by a "learning rule" (Rumelhart et al., 1986). As the network is exposed to stimuli, pathways that transmit signals more often attain higher conduction values. The "memory" of the net is instantiated in the matrix of conduction values or "weights" that hold across the system for the total input set. The hidden units allow the network to attain internal representations. Neural nets have a number of properties that differ from conventional computers. Distributed neural network models are massively redundant. Representation is distributed; damage to the network will reduce resolution or accuracy, but the breakdown is gradual and graded. Unlike a discrete system in which memory is local, damage to some discrete part of the network won't, for example, destroy memory of grandmother's face (Kohonen, 1984). The distributed, redundant computational process exemplified in neural networks appear to be the best present approximations to neural computation. However, the studies discussed in the following chapters show that the human brain is not a single large unitary neural network. Particular neuroanatomical structures are specialized to effect certain types of processes.

Both rules and representations are coded in a similar manner in neural networks. Therefore, many of the linguistic debates regarding the utility of rules versus representations are irrelevant when information is represented in a neural network. Statistical regularities that can be represented as "rules" will emerge as the network is exposed to a set of exemplars. Learning involves structural change, the modification of synaptic weights that build up a representation of rule-governed processes in the network's hidden layers. As recent data demonstrate, human children likewise make use of robust, statistically driven, associative learning to "acquire" the syllabic structure of words (Saffran et al., 1996) and syntax (Singleton and Newport, 1989).

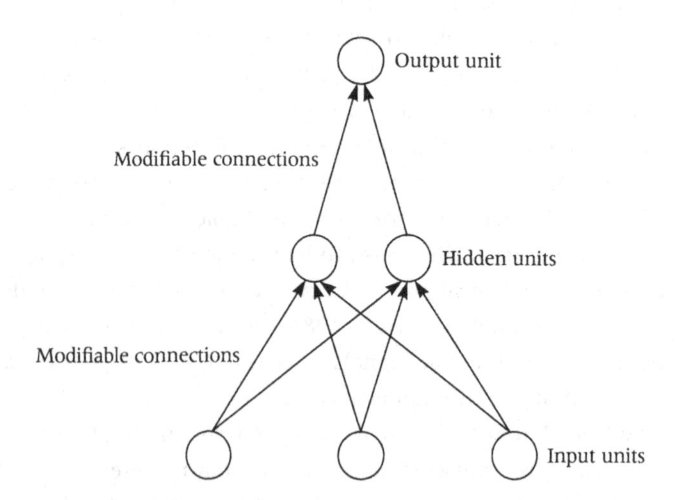

Figure 1-2. A schematic multilayered network. The "hidden units" allow these networks to form internal representations. Multilayer networks of this sort have been shown to approximate various aspects of behavior. (After Bates and Elman, 1993.)

Cortical Maps

It is evident that the human brain (or the brain of any other animal) is not a large amorphous neural network. Different parts of the brain have different *cytoarchitectonic structures,* that is, different types of neurons. The cytoarchitectural maps of brains made by the neuroanatomist Korbinian Brodmann (1908, 1909, 1912) generally appear to reflect functional distinctions. Certain areas of the cortex, such as area 17 in Figure 1–3, are implicated in visual perception. Area 17 receives signals from part of the thalamus, which in turn receives signals from the eye. People who lack area 17 are blind. However, area 17 is also active in visual mental imagery (Kosslyn et al., 1999), and many other cortical areas are implicated in vision. Similar relations characterize motor control. Brodmann's area 4, the primary motor cortex, is only part of the complex assemblage of cortical and subcortical neural structures involved in motor control and is active in perceptual and cognitive tasks that refer to or appear to involve internal modeling of motor activity. Many details remain unknown. The situation is similarly complex and unclear for language. The chapters that follow will demonstrate that subcortical structures play a crucial part in regulating human language. Although Broca's area, which consists of Brodmann's areas 44 and 45 in the dominant, usually left hemisphere of the cortex, is usually implicated in language, children whose entire left hemisphere has been surgically removed don't completely lose the ability to acquire language (Elman et al., 1996; Bates, Vicari, and Trauner, 1999). Broca's and adjacent cortical areas are also implicated in manual motor control (Kimura, 1979, 1993; Krams et al., 1998). And experimental data show that different cortical locations regulate similar aspects of language in the brains of different people (Ojemann and Mateer, 1979; Ojemann et al., 1989). Furthermore, many areas of the cortex can take on new functions after damage to the brain or birth defects (Merzenich et al., 1984; Merzenich, 1987; Sanes and Donoghue, 1994, 1997; Donoghue, 1995; Elman et al., 1996). For example, the visual cortex in humans who were born blind or were blind at an early age appears to be recruited to process tactile perception (Cohen et al., 1997).

Direct Electrophysiologic Recording

Direct observation of neuronal activity in the brain of a living animal involves placing microelectrodes therein. These electrodes conduct electrical signals induced by the electrochemical communications between neurons. In principle, the techniques are similar to those employed by a wiretapper. A small antenna, the microelectrode, is placed in or close to the electrical circuit (the neuronal signal path) that is to be monitored. The microelectrode picks up the signal, which is then amplified and recorded. But whereas a wiretapper can surreptitiously place a miniature antenna close to the circuit connections in a telephone junction box and then remove it without disrupting the telephone system, microelectrode recording techniques are rather invasive.

The microelectrode first has to be driven into the brain of an animal whose skull has been opened. Elaborate precautions must be taken to

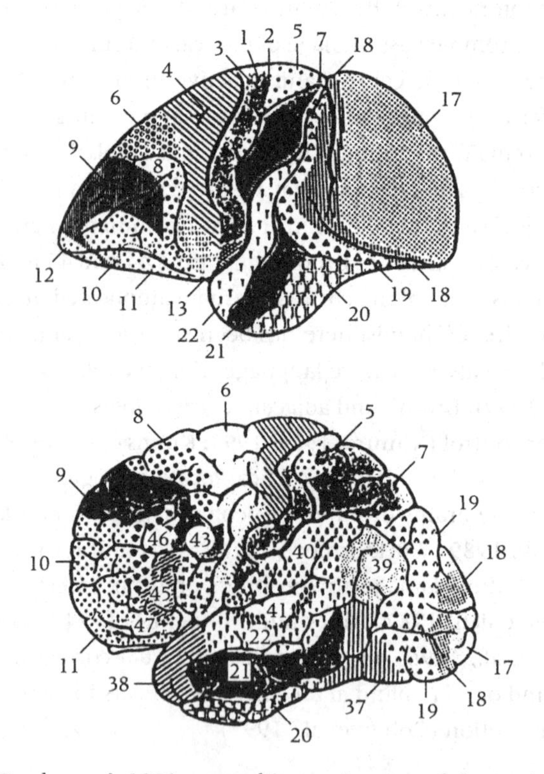

Figure 1-3. Brodmann's 1909 cytoarchitectonic maps of the cortical areas of the macaque monkey (top) and human (bottom) brains. The size of the brains has been equalized here, but the monkey brain's volume is less than one-third that of the human brain. The frontal regions are to the left. Areas 44 and 45 of the human brain are the traditional sites of Broca's area.

achieve useful data. The microelectrode or electrodes first must be positioned in the intended neuroanatomical structure. If the experiment is monitoring neuronal activity connected with the perception or processing of visual, tactile, olfactory, or auditory signals, a representative range of appropriate stimuli must then be presented to the prepared animal. Appropriate motor tasks must be executed by the animal if the focus of the experiment is motor control. Often the interpretation of the cells being monitored is skewed by the range of sensory inputs, motor activities, or the context that was *not* explored. Some of the most revealing studies were serendipitous. For example, the sensory responses of the monkey functional neural system discussed below that seems to be designed to respond to nearby objects would not have been discovered except for the chance event of neuronal activity when a Q-tip happened to be placed close to the eyes of the monkey under study. Finally, the exact positions of the recording electrodes must be determined by sacrificing the experimental animal, sectioning and staining its brain, and examining the stained sections microscopically. In certain limited circumstances, direct electrophysiologic recordings can be made in human patients prior to brain surgery. George Ojemann and his colleagues have obtained many insights into brain function in this manner. However, the range of stimuli, the duration of recording, and the number of locations that can be explored is necessarily limited. Nor can precise electrode placements usually be determined.

Tracer Studies

The technique that reveals the neural circuits regulating various aspects of behavior cannot be used in human subjects. One of the properties of axons is that amino acids, the building blocks of proteins, are transmitted from the cell body down the length of an axon. In the late 1960s it was discovered that radioactively labeled amino acids injected into a cell body are also transported down the axon to its terminal. The pathways from neuron to neuron can then be determined by mapping the radioactive axon terminals. Another tracer technique involves the enzyme horseradish peroxidase (HRP), which has an odd interaction with neurons: it is taken up at the terminal ends of axons and is then transmitted "retrogradely" back to the cell body. Other tracer compounds can be used to map out neuronal circuits. However, all tracer techniques involve injecting substances into the brain of a living animal, waiting for the tracer to be transported, and then sacrificing the animal, sectioning its brain and using chemical reactions to visualize the HRP transport, or other means to map the transport of radioactive tags, and then using microscopic examinations of sliced sections of the animal's brain. Typically "populations," or groups of neurons, "project" (connect) to populations of neurons in other neuroanatomical structures. The circuits usually are "segregated," or anatomically independent. A given neuroanatomical structure typically contains many segregated microcircuits that project to different segregated neuronal populations in other neuroanatomical structures.

Noninvasive Imaging Studies

Although it is impossible to map neuronal circuits in human beings by the invasive techniques described above, noninvasive imaging techniques make it possible to infer neuronal activity associated with various aspects of behavior in human beings. Functional magnetic resonance imaging (fMRI), the most recent of these techniques, is a variant on the structural magnetic resonance imaging (MRI) systems that are routinely used for clinical imaging of brain structures. The basic operating principle involves generating an intense magnetic field which perturbs the electrons of molecular compounds. When the magnetic field is suddenly released, the resetting electrons emit characteristic electromagnetic "signatures," which are mapped by complex computer algorithms. Structural MRI can map "slices" of the brain; fMRI can map out the flow and transport of oxygenated blood and other indirect markers of metabolic activity, hence neural activity, in the brain.

Positron emission tomography (PET), another imaging technique, involves injecting a low dose of a short-half-life radioactive tracer into the bloodstream. Blood flow increases as metabolic activity increases in the parts of the brain active in some task. Radioactively tagged glucose also can be injected into the bloodstream. A computer system then interprets the signals picked up by sensors that monitor the level or amount of the tagged blood or glucose. In essence, both PET and fMRI attempt to follow metabolic activity of various parts of the brain while a person thinks, talks, and so on. The noisiness of fMRI systems limits their use in studies of speech perception. On the other hand, PET involves some exposure to ionizing radiation.

One point that must be kept in mind when interpreting the data and the conclusions of many PET and fMRI studies is the inherent limitation of the "subtractive" technique that is usually applied. A neophrenological cast often implicitly structures many PET and fMRI studies. PET and fMRI experiments using the subtractive technique often assume that activity in a particular location of the brain means that this part of the brain is the "seat" of some aspect of behavior. The pattern of metabolic activity associated with a presumed "baseline" condition is subtracted from the total metabolic pattern associated with the experimental stimuli. For example, activity noted when a person listens to acoustic "white noise" is subtracted from that which occurs when that person listens to words. The net result could be assumed to be the activity of the part of the brain that interprets words. This assumption would overlook the fact that circuits carry out complex behaviors. The neuroanatomical structures implicated in listening to acoustic signals must necessarily be activated when we interpret words. And there is no guarantee that the part of the brain that is supposedly the "seat" of word comprehension is not also activated in other behaviors not explored in the particular experiment.

Overreliance on the subtractive technique sometimes results in breathless press releases announcing the part of the brain that determines some newsworthy aspect of human behavior such as sex, fear, aggression, or loathing. Jerome Kagan's parody of locating the "seat" of tennis by subtracting PET brain activity when thinking about running, from brain activity while thinking about tennis is not too far off the mark when evaluating the claims of some PET and fMRI studies. As we shall see, neuroanatomical structures that are activated in one activity in a particular experiment are generally activated in other behaviors, sometimes closely related, sometimes not.

Computerized tomography (CT) ushered in the modern period of brain research. CT scans differ from conventional X rays (radiographs) in that they show slices of brain anatomy reconstructed by computer processing of multiple X-ray exposures taken at different angles and planes. This technology makes it possible to determine the site and extent of damage in a living patient. MRIs provide better images. One problem in interpreting brain function common to all of these procedures (CT, PET, and fMRI) involves comparing activity in different people's brains. It is clear that people's brains differ as much as faces, feet, hearts, teeth, and other aspects of anatomy (Ojemann et al., 1989; Ziles et al., 1995; Fink et al.). In fact, recent fMRI studies of identical twins by Mazziotta at UCLA show variations even in gyral morphology, reflecting variations in the gross proportions of different parts of their brains.

Event-related potentials (ERPs) provide a complementary technique to both PET and fMRI imaging data. PET and fMRI can determine metabolic activity in a particular part of the brain, but temporal response times are sluggish. The metabolic activity recorded by these techniques represents neural activity averaged over many seconds. ERPs can reveal transient electrical activity recorded by means of electrodes placed in contact with a person's skull. The technique involves recording by means of the EEG procedures commonly used to record brain activity in clinical settings. The difference is that a particular stimulus, for example a spoken word, is presented many times. The electrical signals recorded in response to the stimulus are then summed and averaged. ERPs lack topographic resolution, but they complement the slow temporal resolution of PET and fMRI data.

Experiments in Nature

The study of brain function and theories concerning the neural bases of human language began long before it was possible to perform electrophysiologic, tracer, or imaging studies. Theories tried to account for data derived from studies of behavioral deficits either induced by deliberate lesions in the brains of experimental animals or deduced from the "experiments in nature" that occur when particular parts of a person's brain have been destroyed by accidents, gunshots, strokes, tumors, or other pathologies. Since only human beings possess language, the study of the brain bases of language relied on language deficits, aphasia, induced by experiments in nature. Although the interpretation of the behavioral deficits of aphasia that will be presented in the next chapter is quite different from Paul Broca's (1861) model, experiments in nature are still germane to the brain-language question, particularly when they complement the data of noninvasive imaging studies of neurologically intact subjects.

Functional Neural Systems for Motor Control and Vision

The invasive techniques that would map out the circuits of the FLS obviously cannot be applied to explore human linguistic ability. However, the basic "computational" structure of the human brain clearly is similar to other biological brains by virtue of its evolutionary history. It did not spring forth *de novo*. Therefore, it is appropriate to draw on comparative studies of the brain circuitry that regulates various aspects of motor control and of visual, auditory, and tactile perception in other species. I shall use the term "functional neural system" to describe a network of neural circuits that work together to affect an overt behavior that contributes to the biological fitness of a living creature, that is, some activity that contributes to its survival and the survival of its progeny. The human FLS is a functional neural system that is a derived property of *Homo sapiens.*

Some of the most striking evidence for functional neural systems comes from studies that monitor electrophysiologic activity in the brains of monkeys. These experiments show that a class of functional systems exist that rapidly integrate sensory, cognitive, and motor activity to achieve particular motoric responses to external stimuli. These functional neural systems appear to facilitate the performance of tasks that contribute to an animal's survival and biological fitness.

For example, studies of the brains of monkeys show that functional neural systems have evolved to cope with particular aspects of life involving vision. If we were to follow principles of logic and parsimony that structure philosophic conceptions of "modularity" (Fodor, 1983), it would be reasonable to propose that a single map exists in some part of the brain (presumably in the visual cortex), which other neural modules that regulate hand movements, identifying objects, walking, and so on can reference. The traditional view, now known to be incorrect, of the neural basis of the representation of visual space in the brain was that some part of the visual cortex contains a "map" of space analogous to the representation of a scene in a photograph. Many aspects of behavior depend on visual information, such as moving one's hand toward an object, identifying a particular animal, or avoiding walking over a cliff. All of these activities could involve reference to a single common topographic "map" that codes the location of everything that you see at a given moment.

However, neurophysiologists who study vision conclude that no single, unified, visual "map" exists in the primate brain. Instead, different functional systems exist each of which achieves particular goals. One system explored by Charles Gross and his colleagues (1995) appears to be adapted to grasping or deflecting objects that are moving toward a monkey's face. Their studies of the macaque monkey *(Macaca fasicularis)* brain show that cells in the putamen, a subcortical basal ganglia structure, respond vigorously when a monkey sees small objects approaching its face and eyes. These putamenal neurons do not respond to images, stationary objects, or moving objects more than a meter or so from the monkey. About 25 percent of these sites also respond to tactile sensations on the monkey's face. These putamenal neurons, in turn, communicate to neurons in the monkey's ventral premotor neocortex. In an earlier study Gross and his colleagues showed that many neurons in the ventral premotor cortex respond both to visual stimuli near the monkey's arm or hand and to tactile responses:

> these visual neurons also respond to tactile stimuli; they have tactile receptive fields (RFs) on the face or arms, and corresponding visual RFs extend outward from the tactile fields into the space surrounding the body. The tactile fields are somatotopically organized, and therefore the corresponding visual RFs provide a map of visual space near the body . . . a population of these cells could specify the location of targets for limb and body movements. (Graziano et al., 1994, p. 1054)

In other words, the visual responses of these neurons are arm-centered; they provide a representation of space near the body that is useful for grasping objects moving toward the monkey. This functional close-object-intercept system directly links inputs from the visual cortex and tactile inputs to the putamen, premotor cortex, motor cortex, and the monkey's arms and hands, integrating sight, touch, and muscular control to achieve a specific task—intercepting objects. It doesn't require an ethological study of monkeys in their natural habitat to predict that individuals who can better avoid being hit in the head or eyes will be more likely to survive and produce more descendants. It also is obvious that the system is not organized along logical, "parsimonious," modular principles. Although specialized areas of the cortex process incoming visual information, no general-purpose "visual module" exists that processes all visual input and then sends appropriate vectors to a "motor interception module." Nor does an independent "tactile-perception" module exist.

Other electrophysiologic studies show that the primary motor cortex of monkeys is also organized in a functional manner. The traditional view of the primary motor cortex was a "somatopic" map of an animal's body that charted a one-to-one correspondence between specific cortical areas and the parts of the body that they supposedly controlled. Individual muscles were supposedly activated by particular cortical neurons; for example, the thumb was controlled by neurons in one area, the fingers by neurons in another, and the wrist in a pattern that mirrored the shape of the hand. Many texts still represent the organization of the human primary motor cortex by means of an upside-down cartoon of the body (toes, feet, hand, fingers, lips, tongue, etc.) in which different areas of the motor cortex control a given part of the body. However, a series of studies (reviewed in Barinaga, 1995) that started in the late 1970s shows that individual muscles are influenced by neurons in several separate locations in the motor cortex. Moreover, individual cortical neurons have branches linking them to other cortical neurons that control multiple muscles. The complex assemblage of neurons appears to be a functionally organized system in which circuits consisting of neuronal populations work together to coordinate groups of muscles that carry out particular actions.

Recent data on the human primary motor cortex are consistent with the monkey data noted above. The data obtained by Sanes et al. (1995) using functional magnetic resonance imaging (fMRI) to study human subjects performing motor tasks are similar to those studied in monkeys using invasive techniques. Multiple representations, circuits, and controlling finger and wrist movements in the human primary motor cortex were charted during different voluntary movements. As Sanes and his colleagues note, the hypothesis that best explains their data is one in which "neurons within the M1 [primary motor cortex] arm area form a distributed and cooperative network that can simultaneously and optimally control collections of arm muscles . . . Furthermore, it is likely that neural elements or ensembles that make up the functional processing units continually recombine while forming new output properties to produce normal adaptive behavior" (p. 1777).

Although data on speech motor activity are not available, it is unlikely that the role of the primary motor cortex in speech differs from other aspects of motor control. The organization of the primary motor cortex is not somatopically "modular," although general regions of the primary motor cortex control head, arm, and leg movements. Discrete areas controlling fingers, wrist, tongue, and lips do not exist.

Diffuse neuronal populations instead appear to be shaped to regulate learned motor control patterns (Donoghue, 1995; Karni et al., 1995, 1998; Pascual-Leone et al., 1995: Sanes et al., 1995; Nudo et al., 1996; Sanes and Donoghue, 1996, 1997, in press; Classen et al., 1998). The potential for the neural control of complex motor activity is part of the genotype. The circuits that regulate particular movements in animals and humans are not necessarily genetically specified. Many are formed as an individual animal learns to perform a particular task. They reflect the end result of the process of "automatization" by which means animals, including humans, learn to rapidly execute skilled "motor control programs" (MCPs) without conscious thought. In fact the primary motor cortex appears to be adapted for learning and storing these MCPs (Evarts, 1973). Repeated trials appear to shape neuronal circuits. The process is apparent when a novice driver learns to shift the gears of a car that has a manual transmission. At first shifting requires total concentration and is slow and inaccurate. After repeated trials, gear-shifting becomes automatic and rapid. Similar effects occur as we "learn" to walk, catch balls, or talk.

CHAPTER 2

Speech Production and Perception

Since speech is central to the proposed functional language system, it is necessary to take note of the nature of speech production and speech perception, as well as the general role of speech in the FLS, particularly with reference to lexical access and the comprehension of distinctions in meaning deriving from syntax.

Neural Regulation

The traditional Broca's–Wernicke's areas theory for the brain bases of language localizes speech production to "the third frontal convolution" of the neocortex. But imaging studies of neurologically intact subjects reveal a more complex picture. For example, the PET study of Peterson et al. (1988), in which neurologically intact subjects were asked either to read or to repeat isolated spoken words, showed activation of the primary motor cortex, the premotor cortex, and the supplementary motor cortex in the subjects' left hemispheres and bilateral activation of areas near Broca's area and its right-hemisphere homologue. Bilateral activation of areas near Broca's region also occurred when subjects were asked simply to move their mouths and tongues. This finding is consistent, to a degree, with the data from many studies of patients having cortical lesions since lesions confined to Broca's area often result in oral apraxia, deficits in motor control instead of the deficits in motor planning associated with aphasia (Kimura, 1979, 1993; Stuss and Benson, 1986).

However, imaging studies show that the neural basis of speech production is not restricted to the premotor and motor cortex, Broca's area, or even the frontal regions of the brain. A series of PET studies performed at the Montreal Neurological Institute has consistently shown increased activity in

Brodmann's areas 47, 46, 45, and 8 in the left frontal region as well as activity in the subcortical left putamen and the posterior secondary "auditory" cortex. These studies demonstrate the presence of pathways from "motor" to "auditory" cortex. Signals transmitted from neural structures regulating speech motor control result in increased activity in regions of the posterior temporal cortex associated with speech perception when a person talks (Klein et al., 1994, 1995; Paus, 1996). Masking noise was used in these experiments to prevent the subjects from hearing themselves, so the increased activity cannot be ascribed to an auditory input. Increased neuronal activity in regions of the auditory cortex associated with speech perception has been noted in tasks that involve auditory imagery (Zatorre et al., 1996) and inner speech and silent reading (Paulesu, Firth, and Frackowiak, 1993; Bavelier et al., 1995), congruent with the activation of the visual cortex in mental imagery (Kosslyn et al., 1999) noted earlier.

Other types of data also indicate a wider locus of cortical sites implicated in speech production and other aspects of language than would be expected if the traditional Lichtheim (1885) model were correct. In studies spanning many years, Ojemann and his colleagues electrically stimulated areas of the cortex exposed before surgery in awake subjects. Subjects had difficulty producing sequential orofacial articulatory maneuvers when locations in or near the region usually identified as Broca's area were stimulated (Ojemann and Mateer, 1979). However, Ojemann and his colleagues also mapped locations in or near Broca's region at which *both* the production of sequential orofacial movements and the perception of consonant-vowel segments were disrupted. Subjects also produced agrammatic utterances with low-voltage electrical stimulation at some of these sites. Many of the stimulation sites were posterior to Broca's area and differed from subject to subject. Interference with speech perception, which is significant in the light of the "motor theory of speech perception" discussed below, also occurred at some of these sites.

The Ojemann group's data also suggest that the neuronal processes supported in these sites are not genetically specified, but are instead acquired phenotypically in a manner similar to the neural bases of various aspects of motor control (e.g., Karni et al., 1995, 1998; Nudo et al., 1996; Pascual-Leone et al., 1995; Sanes et al., 1995; Classen et al., 1998). The group studied 117 patients, using the stimulation technique to locate cortical sites at which the ability to name objects was interrupted (Ojemann et al., 1989). The location at which this occurred varied dramatically from subject to subject, spreading over a large region of posterior temporal regions of the cortex. Stimulation of cortical sites far removed from Wernicke's area interfered with subjects' ability to name objects.

Physiology of Speech Production

"Motor equivalence" characterizes the ability of animals and humans to accomplish the same goal using different muscles or different body parts. Motor equivalence is apparent when you write your name by holding a pencil between your teeth instead of your fingers. It is also apparent when the electrical activity of the cortex is monitored while human subjects perform the deceptively simple task of flexing their index finger on the beat of a metronome. Different patterns of neural activity that yielded motor equivalence were apparent even as subjects performed this task (Kelso et al., 1998). Converging evidence shows that the production of human speech is a supreme example of motor equivalence directed toward achieving distal acoustic goals. Competent human speakers have at their command families of alternate motor control "programs" that coordinate different groups of muscles to produce a particular speech sound. It is also apparent that the perception of speech is in a meaningful sense "special." Motoric aspects of speech production form part of the information set that we use to perceive the sounds of speech (Liberman et al., 1967; Lindblom, 1996).

Some background information on the physiology of human speech production may be useful at this point. Human speech results from the activity of three functionally distinct systems: (1) the subglottal lungs, (2) the larynx, and (3) the supralaryngeal airway—the supralaryngeal vocal tract (SVT). The acoustic consequences of the physiology of these systems have been studied since the early nineteenth century, when Johannes Müller (1848) formulated what has come to be known as the "source-filter" theory of speech production. Figure 2-1 shows the anatomy involved in the production of human speech.

Müller noted that the outward flow of air from the lungs usually provides the power for speech production. If the human auditory system were capable of perceiving acoustic energy at extremely low frequencies, we would "hear" the expiratory airflow. However, the acoustic energy present in the outward flow of air from the lungs is inaudible. Two different sources of acoustic energy enter into the production of human speech: periodic *phonation* and/or turbulent *noise*. *Phonation* results from laryngeal activity. The vocal folds (or cords; the two terms refer to the same structures) of the larynx, which are extremely complex structures, move inward and outward, converting the steady flow of air flowing outward from the lungs into a series of "puffs" of air. Both the basic rate and the pattern of airflow through the phonating larynx can be modulated by adjusting the tension of the laryngeal muscles and the alveolar air pressure generated by the lungs. The *fundamental frequency of phonation,* F0, is the rate at which the vocal folds open and close. The perceptual response of human listeners to F0 is the *pitch* of a speaker's voice. Young children have high F0s; their voices are therefore perceived as "high pitched." Adult males usually have lower F0s and the pitch of their voices is low. The larynx is an efficient energy transducer, converting the inaudible airflow from the lungs into a rich source of audible sound energy; the puffs of air produced during phonation yield acoustic energy at F0 and the harmonics of the F0. For example, if F0 is 100 Hz, energy can occur at 200 Hz, 300 Hz, 400 Hz, and so on. The amplitude of the

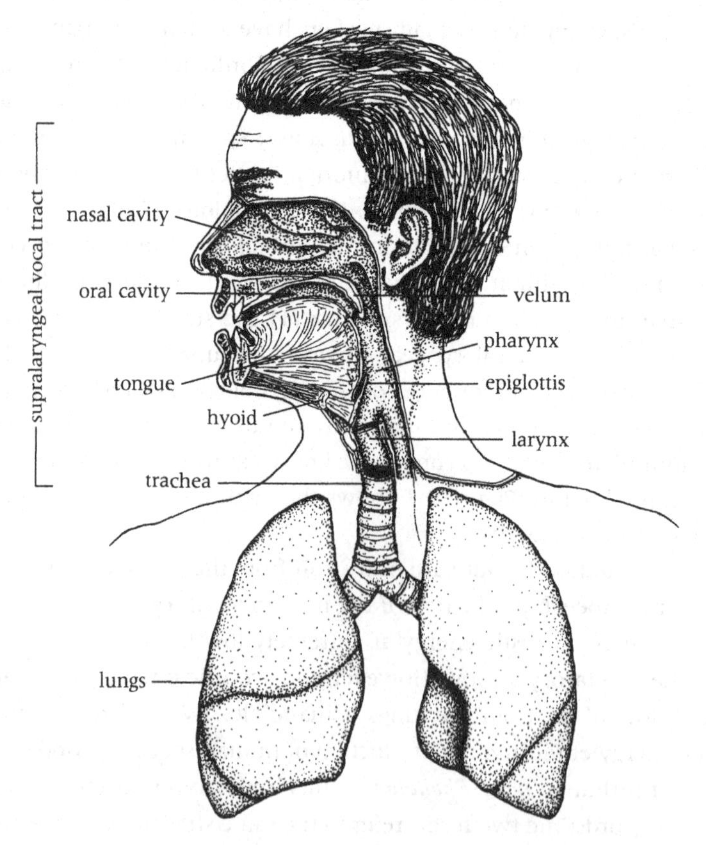

Figure 2-1. The anatomy involved in the production of human speech.

energy produced at each harmonic gradually falls off at higher frequencies, but the net result is the production of acoustic energy at many audible frequencies.

Noise sources are aperiodic and usually have acoustic energy evenly distributed across all audible frequencies. Noise sources can be generated by turbulent airflow at constrictions along the airway leading out from the trachea. Noise generated at the larynx by forcing air through the partly abducted vocal cords forms the source of acoustic energy for the consonant [h] at the start of the word *hat*. The noise sources for other consonants are generated by forcing air through constrictions higher in the SVT. For example, the initial consonant of the word *shoe* is generated at the constriction formed by the tongue blade raised close to the hard palate of the mouth. The initial noise burst of the stop consonant [t] of the word *to* is generated when the tongue "releases" the occlusion of the SVT, moving away from the hard palate. The burst is momentary because the turbulent noise abruptly ceases when the airflow changes from turbulent to laminar flow as the tongue blade moves farther away from the palate.

Other linguistic distinctions rest on temporal factors. The distinction between the English stop consonants [b] and [p] when they occur in syllable-initial position, for example, rests on the sequential timing between the release-burst that occurs when the speaker's lips open and the onset of phonation. The sound [b] is produced when phonation occurs near in time to the release of the burst, [p] when phonation is delayed. This phonetic distinction, "voice-onset time" (VOT), the elapsed time between release-burst and phonation onset, appears to be common to all human languages (Lisker and Abramson, 1964); it differentiates sounds such as [d] from [t] and [g] from [k] in English. "Voiced" stop consonants such as [b], [d], and [g] are produced with a short VOT, "unvoiced" stop consonants such as [p], [t], and [k] with long VOTs.[1] VOT necessitates controlling the sequence in which independent articulatory structures, the larynx and the lips or tongue, perform gestures. When speakers fail to regulate VOT properly and produce VOTs for stop consonants such as [b] and [p] that overlap or fail to maintain a 20-msec separation, it becomes difficult to perceive their intentions. The sound [b] may be perceived as a [p] or [p] as [b]. VOT deficits are one of the distinguishing features of Broca's aphasia, Parkinson's disease, and other conditions in which subcortical components of the FLS circuits are compromised.

However, the acoustic cues produced by the modulation of the supralaryngeal vocal tract's shape are arguably the primary characteristics of human speech. As Müller (1848) pointed out, the acoustic energy that is produced by the larynx is necessarily filtered by the airway above the larynx. The same consideration applies to noise sources; the acoustic energy is filtered by the airway above the constriction at which noise is generated. What we hear is the result of the supralaryngeal airway acting as an acoustic filter.

The frequencies at which maximum energy passes through the airway acting as a filter are called *formant frequencies*. The physiology of speech is in this regard analogous to a harmonica. The immediate source of acoustic energy for the harmonica is its diaphragm, which produces periodic "puffs" of air. The harmonica's tubes act as acoustic filters, transmitting maximum acoustic energy at their "formants." The note that we perceive at any moment reflects the formant frequency determined by a particular tube length. As the musician plays the harmonica, unstopping different tubes, the formants change; the term "resonance" is usually used to describe this effect in musical instruments. The process may perhaps be easier to "see" if one thinks of the view of the world that is presented when we wear sunglasses. The sunglasses act as a filter, absorbing electromagnetic energy at certain frequencies. At other frequencies, which determine the color of the sunglasses, maximum energy passes through. The sunglasses can filter light that intrinsically has different degrees of energy at different frequencies, such as candlelight and sunlight. However, the inherent color of the sunglasses is a characteristic of the dyes used to determine the filtering effects of the glasses. One can wear blue-, amber-, or red-tinted sunglasses.

The human supralaryngeal vocal tract is essentially a tube whose shape and length can be continually modified as we move our lower jaw, tongue body, tongue blade, lips, larynx, and velum. The velum can open or close our nose, thereby coupling a second tube into the system. The phonetic quality of the "segmental" sounds of speech is largely determined by their formant frequency patterns. The vowel sound [i], the vowel of the word *bee* (the brackets signify "phonetic" notation) is signaled by a particular *pattern* of formant frequencies F1, F2, F3. For a male speaker having a supralaryngeal vocal tract length of 17 cm, F1 = 0.3 kHz, F2 = 2.1 kHz, F3 = 3.1 kHz. The same speaker's [u] vowel, the vowel of the word *boo,* would have an F1 = 0.35 kHz, F2 = 0.8 kHz, F3 = 2.2 kHz. As we talk we continually adjust the positions of our tongue, velum (which can seal the nasal cavity), lips, jaw, and larynx to produce SVT configurations that yield the formant frequency patterns of each sound.

The formant frequency patterns of particular speech sounds derive from particular SVT configurations. Because we cannot move these anatomical structures with infinite speed, the SVT configuration must gradually shift from the SVT configuration of one speech sound to that of the next speech sound. As the supralaryngal vocal tract configuration gradually changes so do the formant frequencies. The result is an acoustic melding in which the formant patterns that specify "individual" sounds are "encoded" into syllable-sized units (Liberman et al., 1967). For example, it is impossible to produce the isolated sound [b] without also producing some vowel or "continuant" such as [ba] or [bs]. This process yields the high information transfer rate of human speech; the rate at which speech sounds can be transmitted (20 to 30 phonetic units per second) exceeds the fusion frequency of the human auditory system. The acoustic cues that convey speech are encoded into syllable-sized units whose transmission rate does not exceed the fusion frequency of the auditory system. The encoded syllables then can be resolved into the phonetic code.

The "motor theory of speech perception" proposed by Alvin Liberman (1967) and his colleagues at Haskins Laboratories proposed that the decoding process entailed resolving the acoustic signal into the invariant articulatory patterns that hypothetically generated the formant frequency pattern of each phonetic element, such as the [c], [ae], and [t] of the word *cat.* However, the situation is more complex; different people use different motor control patterns to achieve the "same" acoustic goal. For example, Terrance Nearey's (1979) cineradiographic study of three speakers of American English all of whom were specialists in acoustic phonetics showed that each produced the same vowels using different vocal tract configurations. One person hardly moved his tongue (traditional phonetic theories postulate different tongue positions for different vowels); he instead generated different appropriate formant frequency patterns by adjusting the position of his lips and larynx. Other radiographic studies of vowel production yielded similar results (Russell, 1928; Carmody, 1937; Ladefoged et al., 1972).

As noted earlier, motor equivalence characterizes many aspects of human and animal behavior. Motor equivalence allows human speakers to produce well-formed speech when "normal" speaking conditions are disrupted, without any special instructions or tutoring. This can easily be demonstrated if you place your index finger atop one of your teeth and talk. Although the normal movements of the jaw are impeded, you will automatically compensate for the fact that you cannot close your jaw and will produce normal formant frequency patterns by means of alternate motor commands. The process is in place by age three years. Experimental data show that children as young as age three-years produce the formant frequency patterns of vowels with their "normal" values when speaking with 10 mm high-bite blocks. The children move their tongues higher than normal when producing the vowels [i] or [u], which are normally produced by moving the lower jaw upward. In other words, they compensate for the reduced mobility of their lower jaws by moving their tongues higher. This compensatory process occurs without auditory feedback, since at no time do they produce the inappropriate formant frequency patterns that would result if they had not compensated for lower-jaw immobility (Baum and Katz, 1984). The neurally coded motor control "programs" that govern this process may reflect the effects of learning to talk at an early age with food and/or other objects in one's mouth.

The motor command sequences that underlie the production of human speech are arguably the most complex that ordinary people attain. Some notion of the complexity of the automatized motor control patterns that underlie human speech may be gained by looking at experimental data. Gracco and Abbs (1985) devised an experiment in which a small electrical servomotor could abruptly apply a force to a speaker's lower lip, impeding its closing. The speakers were asked to produce a series of syllables that started with the sound [b]. The stop consonant [b] is produced by closing one's lips. The experimenters first used the motor to occasionally impede lip closing 40 msec before the point when they would have normally reached a closed position. The speakers compensated for the perturbation within 40 msec and closed their lips by applying more muscle force to their lower lip. The speakers also helped close their lips with a slight downward movement of their upper lips. The experimenters found that the speakers needed a minimum time of 40 msec to perform these compensating maneuvers. This interval corresponds to the time that it takes for a sensory signal to travel up to the motor cortex and a compensating muscular control signal to travel back to the lips (Evarts, 1973). The experimenters then shortened the time between the perturbing force and normal lip closure to 20 msec. The speakers then compensated with a large downward upper-lip deflection, prolonging the duration of the lip closure an additional 20 msec so that there would be sufficient time to overcome the perturbing force by means of lower lip action. The speakers used two different automatized motor response patterns that had a common linguistic goal—closing the lips to produce the consonantal stop closure. The speakers' FLSs must have had a neural representation of a linguistic goal, closing one's lips for a [b], that can be realized by alternate articulatory maneuvers.

The point that is germane here is that motor equivalence characterizes the production of speech sounds. The results of many independent studies (see Lieberman and Blumstein, 1988; or Lindblom, 1988, for background material) show that our brains must contain the instruction sets for "families" of motor control "programs" for the muscles of the tongue, lips, jaw, larynx, and velum that generate the same distal acoustic product—the particular formant frequency patterns, phonation or noise sources, and timing sequences that define particular speech-sounds. The process is a special case of "motor equivalence" directed toward the distal goal of similar acoustic signals.

Articulatory versus Auditory Phonetics

Since the goal of linguistic science is to understand how human beings communicate and think by means of language, we must determine the articulatory and acoustic elements of the sound pattern of speech that have *linguistic* significance, and how they are coded in the mind-brain. One central question is whether the code is based on speech production, specifications of the articulatory maneuvers that produce speech sounds, the acoustic cues that characterize differentiate speech sounds, or both articulation and acoustics.

Throughout the nineteenth century one of the central debates of linguistic research was whether articulatory or acoustic descriptions best characterized the sounds of speech. Linguists attempted to describe the historical changes that occur in all human languages. The words of William Shakespeare's English sound quite different from either contemporary British or American English and differed dramatically from Old English. The linguists of the nineteenth century attempted to formulate "laws" governing sound change. The immediate question was whether the observed sound changes could be best characterized by articulatory or acoustic descriptions. For example, it was possible to specify a "recipe" for producing the stop consonant [b] by describing the position of the lips and the activity of the larynx. Alexander Graham Bell (1867), whose primary concern was teaching deaf people to speak, had devised an elaborate system of "visible speech" which specified the presumed articulatory maneuvers that would produce a speech sound.

Bell, of course, was limited by available technology, and his articulatory specifications are often erroneous. However, his system did explain many observed historical sound changes. Words that started with consonants such as [v], in which the tongue tip is elevated toward the front (anterior) roof of the mouth (hard palate) just behind the teeth, were historically related to words in which the tongue assumed a similar position but differed with respect to the activity of the larynx. The sound [v] is produced while the vocal cords of the larynx rapidly open and close, producing "phonation," or "voicing" (the two terms are synonymous). The sound [f], in contrast, is produced with the tongue in about the same position, but the larynx is instead open, resulting in high airflow and turbulent "noise" produced at the tongue-tip-to-palate constriction. The articulatory parameter "place of articulation," which specifies the similar placement of the tongue tip with respect to the palate for [v] and [f], thus explains the close historical relation between the words *vater* and *father* in German and English. The SVT shapes that generate these sounds are quite similar.

As noted earlier, research techniques have a profound effect on theory. Articulatory descriptions of speech sounds were appropriate during a period in which the only way that a sound could be reproduced was by a human speaker attempting to say it aloud. Unfortunately, radiographic studies that reveal the actual movements of the tongue, lips, and other structures of the vocal tract show the traditional articulatory vowel "features" specifying hypothetical tongue positions that date back to Bell (1867) are not useful descriptors for either phonetic or linguistic phonologic analyses. This should not be viewed as a critique of Bell's research skills; he worked without benefit of imaging techniques that reveal the actual position of a speaker's tongue. What is surprising is that Bell's hypothetical articulatory "instructions" for producing particular vowels are still accepted by speech theorists (Liberman and Mattingley, 1985) and linguists (Chomsky and Halle, 1968) as invariant specifications for the sounds of speech. Nearey's (1979) cineradiographic study, for example, demonstrated that Bell's articulatory "recipes" for vowel production do not even characterize the *relationships* between vowels that might explain historical sound changes. For example, the articulatory vowel feature that hypothetically *always* differentiates the vowel [I] of the word *bit* from the vowel [E] of the word *bet* is the "height" of the tongue, which is supposed to be "higher," that is, closer to the palate, for [I] than for [E]. But the tongue is actually higher for [E] than for [I] for one of Nearey's three subjects and identical for another. The different formant frequency patterns that differentiate [I] from [ae] are achieved by the speakers' making subtle changes in the opening and positions of their lips and the larynges. The speakers appear to be aiming at producing particular formant frequency patterns. Nearey demonstrates that the linguistic "affinity" relationships that exist between vowels are defined by their acoustic proximity. In other words, [I] always has a higher F2 than [ae].

Attempts were made early in the history of systematic phonetic studies to describe speech sounds in terms of their acoustic parameters. Voicing was an obvious candidate. The anatomy of the larynx and the general characteristics of the physiology of phonation were known to Johannes Müller (1848). Müller was able to show that certain sounds, such as vowels and consonants like [m], [n], and [v], clearly were voiced. Hellwag in 1781 was able to determine the formant frequencies of the vowels of German. Hellwag's auditory analysis (he matched the notes of a piano to the perceived qualities of vowels) yielded close approximations of the first two formant frequencies, Fl and F2, that differentiate many vowels (Nearey, 1979). Müller (1848) also formulated the modern source-filter theory of speech production (Chiba and Kajiyama, 1941; Fant, 1960) in qualitative terms. He noted that the phonetic quality of voiced speech sounds was a function of both the laryngeal source and the SVT's shape and length. European linguists, particularly those of the "Prague" school (Jakobson, 1940; Jakobson, Fant, and Halle, 1952) continued to describe the sound patterns of different languages in terms of hypothetical acoustic features.

By the 1930s acoustic analytic techniques were becoming available, and the source-filter theory first proposed by Müller was corroborated (Chiba and Kajiyama, 1941; Fant, 1960). Attested acoustic features could be determined that specified particular speech sounds. Radiographic and electromyographic studies were also beginning to provide actual data concerning the articulatory gestures and muscle activity that produced speech sounds. The linguist Roman Jakobson and his colleagues (1952) provided a framework for the acoustic specification of speech sounds, linking acoustic parameters to articulation. However, the two systems appeared to be at odds. Speech must be perceived by ear. There obviously must be acoustic parameters that humans use to identify speech sounds. However, we also talk. Therefore, we must "know" the appropriate articulatory gestures, muscle commands, and so on that are used to generate speech. At some level this information must be integrated.

The Motor Theory of Speech Perception

Motor theories of speech perception were one answer to this question. Traditional motor theories, which date back to the late nineteenth century (discussed by Zhinkin, 1968), claim that a person actually moved her or his tongue, lips, and so on to generate an internalized sound that is compared with an incoming speech-sound. The articulatory gestures that generate the best match between the incoming and internally generated signal are those that specify the speech sound. The motor theory of speech perception proposed by Alvin Liberman and his colleagues at Haskins Laboratories in the 1960s did not claim that overt articulatory maneuvers must occur. Liberman and his colleagues instead proposed that a listener uses a special process, a "speech mode," to perceive speech. The incoming speech signal is hypothetically interpreted by neurally modeling the sequence of articulatory gestures that produces the best match against the incoming signal. The internal "articulatory" representation is the linguistic construct. In other words, we perceive speech by subvocally modeling speech, without producing any overt articulatory movements. Whereas it is difficult to isolate any invariant acoustic cues that specify the individual sounds of speech that we hear, which roughly correspond to the letters of the alphabet, the Haskins Laboratories theory claimed that the motor commands that generated these phonetic segments were invariant.

Some aspects of the Haskins Laboratories motor theory, revised to a degree by Liberman and Mattingly (1985), are supported by robust experimental data. For example, the Haskins theory claims that human speech is perceived in a "speech mode" distinct from other auditory signals. Acoustic details that are seemingly insignificant must be preserved if the signal is to be heard as speech. For example, the vocal cords of the larynx, which rapidly open and close during phonation, produce a "micro" vibrato. The duration of the pitch period (the inverse 1/F0 of F0) varies slightly from one period to the next. These "pitch perturbations," or "jitter" (the two terms are synonymous), typify human speech (Lieberman, 1961). An alternating series of long-short-long-short periods occurs even when we attempt to produce a steady pitch. The degree to which jitter occurs depends on laryngeal pathology and psychological stress (Lieberman, 1963a; Kagan, Reznick, and Snidman, 1988). However, F0 jitter is always present in human speech. When F0 jitter is removed from the speech signal by computer processing (the simplest technique is to replicate a single period using a waveform editor, reduplicating the period to produce a vowel that has a normal duration and unvarying "perfect" pitch), the resulting sound no longer sounds like speech. It instead sounds like a mechanical buzzer, although all other aspects of the speech signal are preserved. The signal has lost one of the defining characteristics of human speech, F0 jitter, and is no longer perceived in the "speech mode."

Liberman et al. (1967), furthermore, showed that the formant frequency transitions that signaled speech sounds were perceived quite differently when isolated from the total acoustic context that typifies a speech signal. Figure 2-2 illustrates the effect. The bars on the plot are the schematized patterns of the first two formant frequencies, F1 and F2, which served as control signals to a speech synthesizer. These two formants are minimal cues that will convey the syllables [di] and [du] respectively. Although fully specified speech contains information in the third formant frequency pattern that specifies these syllables, the artificial speech signals generated by the Haskins Laboratories synthesizer were not atypical of speech communication in many everyday circumstances. Many hearing-impaired persons perceive speech limited to the F1 and F2 frequency range; many telephone systems transmitted signals limited to F1 and F2. Note that the F2 formant transitions at the start of the syllables provide acoustic cues that signal both the different vowels of each syllable and the "same" [d] consonant. The F2 formant transition rises for [di] and falls for [du] because it is inherently impossible to produce the sound [d] without producing some "continuant," usually a vowel before or after it. The human brain "knows" this, perceiving the two formant transitions as cues for the "same" speech sound, [d], presumably by means of some process that involves internalized knowledge of speech production. This represents the "encoding" process that yields the high data transmission of speech. The encoded syllable is decoded into the speech sounds [d] and [i] or [u]. When human listeners are presented with these same formant transitions in a manner that places them outside the "speech mode," the two formant frequency patterns are instead heard as either ascending or descending "chirps." This can be done by means of computer synthesis in which the two formant frequency transitions are isolated from their steady-state F2 patterns and the similar F1 patterns.

Computer models have successfully determined the formant frequencies of vowels by comparing the incoming acoustic signal to the product of an internal model of the supralaryngeal vocal tract excited by a periodic source (Bell et al., 1961). The Liberman et al. (1967) theory, in essence, reduces to a similar model. A listener hypothetically interprets an incoming speech signal by comparing the products of a neural model constrained by the speech-production constraints of the human supralaryngeal vocal tract. The neural model computes the acoustic consequences of a range of possible articulatory gestures; it selects the articulatory gesture that generates the closest match with the incoming acoustic signal. However, as noted earlier, motor equivalence also argues against any motor theory of speech perception that derives invariant articulatory gestures that hold across all human speakers. Radiographic studies of speech production have consistently shown that different speakers may produce the "same" speech sound using different articulatory gestures (e.g., Russell, 1928; Carmody, 1937; Ladefoged et al. 1972; Nearey, 1979). Nearey's cineradiographic study of vowel production, for example, showed that three phonetically trained members of the

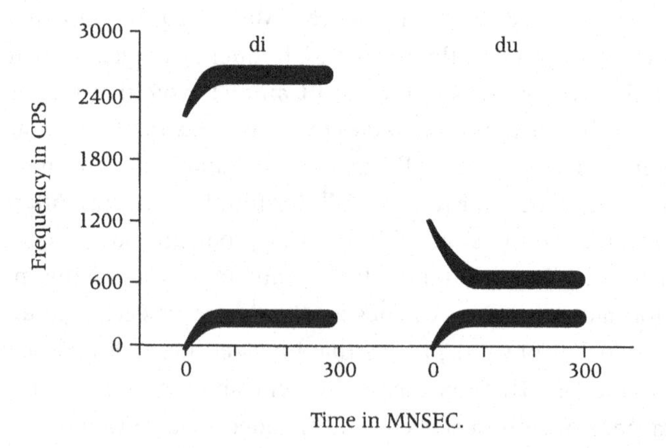

Figure 2-2. When these two stylized formant frequency plots are used to control an appropriate speech synthesizer, the syllables [di] and [du] will be produced.

Haskins Laboratories research staff used different SVT shapes when they carefully spoke the same vowels of English.

Vocal Tract Normalization and Speech Perception

It is clear that any motor theory of speech perception must take account of another obvious aspect of human anatomy. Human beings differ with respect to length of their supralaryngeal vocal tracts (SVTs). For example, children obviously have shorter vocal tracts than adults, and the vocal tracts of adults differ in length. Vocal tract length, in itself, will yield different formant frequencies for the same speech sound (Peterson and Barney, 1952; Fant, 1960; Nearey, 1979). A person internally modeling the incoming acoustic speech signal produced by a vocal tract that has a different length from his own somehow has to take this into account. An adult, for example, cannot physically produce the formant frequency patterns generated by a five-year-old's shorter SVT. Nor could the child produce the adult SVT's formant frequencies. Therefore, any internal modeling of incoming acoustic speech signals by some neural instantiation of an articulatory-gesture-to-acoustic-signal process must deal with SVT normalized signals.

Nearey's (1979) cineradiographic study of vowel production could be interpreted as a claim that speech perception involves only acoustic factors, that any consideration of speech articulation or supralaryngeal vocal tract morphology is not germane to the perception of speech. However, Nearey also complemented his study of vowel production with perceptual experiments. Nearey (1979) showed that human listeners take into account the constraints imposed by the SVT when they perceive speech. Figure 2-3 shows the averaged F1 and F2 values of the vowels produced in words having the form hVd (*had, hid, heed,* etc.) as measured by Peterson and Barney (1952) for a large sample of adult males, adult females, and adolescents. As expected, formant frequency values are transposed upward as average SVT length decreases in much the same manner as shorter organ pipes yield notes that have higher frequencies than those produced by longer pipes.

Note that the formant frequencies of different vowels produced by speakers having shorter or longer SVTs can overlap, The [a]s produced by adult males, for example, have about the same average F1 and F2 values as the [c]s produced by the adolescent children. Many psychoacoustic experiments have confirmed Hellwag's (1781) theory that F1 and F2 provide sufficient information for human listeners to identify a vowel. Speech synthesizers that generate only these two formants produce acceptable vowels (Fant, 1860). However, a computer that was programmed to recognize vowels from their F1 and F2 values would not be able to place an "overlap" stimulus into the proper phonetic category unless it had some knowledge of whether the SVT that generated the signal were that of an adolescent or an adult male. Nearey demonstrated that a computer program could appropriately place the raw F1, F2 Peterson and Barney (1952) data into the appropriate phonetic category if the computer first "heard" an [i] vowel formant pattern. The formant patterns corresponding to [i]s never overlap. Thus any

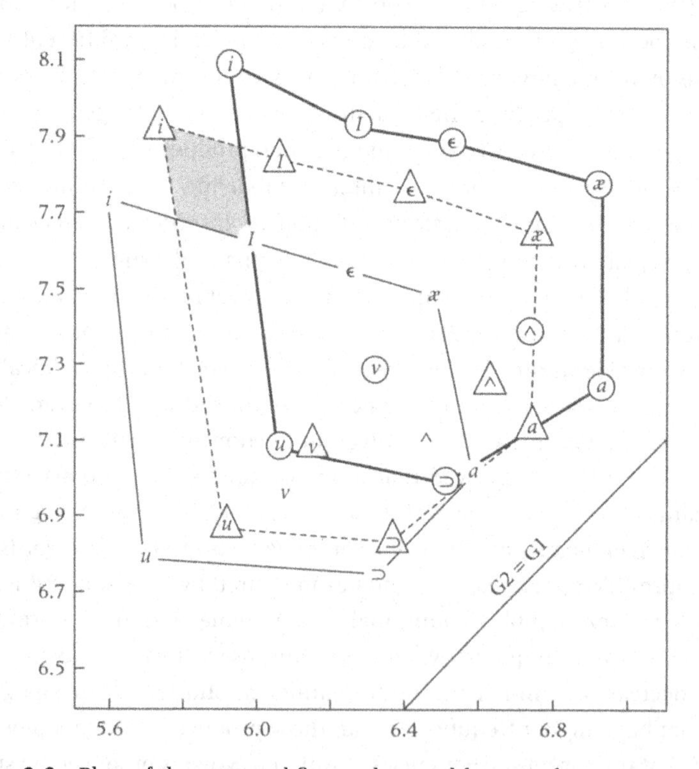

Figure 2-3. Plots of the averaged first and second formant frequency combinations that specify the vowels of English for the men, women, and adolescents studied by Peterson and Barney (1952). Nearey replotted these average values of F1 and F2 on a logarithmic scale. The shape of the plots is similar; they are simply transposed in frequency because the vocal tracts of men, women, and children differ in length. (After Nearey, 1978.)

F1, F2 pattern that specifies an [i] automatically identifies itself. Figure 2-3 shows the nonoverlap of [i]s along the extreme upper left of the vowel space diagrams.

Moreover, whereas many other vowels can be and are generated by means of alternate articulatory maneuvers, the human SVT is constrained to one particular configuration that is necessary to produce the combination of formant frequencies that specify an [i] vowel (Stevens and House, 1955). The tongue body is positioned as high as possible, to the point where air turbulence would occur if it came closer to the palate, and as far front as possible; lip protrusion is minimized, and the larynx is positioned high (Fant, 1960; Stevens, 1972; Perkell and Nelson, 1982, 1985; Beckman et al., 1995; Story, Titze, and Hoffman, 1996). The degree of constriction for [i] is also stabilized because of a physiological "saturation" effect (Fujimura and Kakita, 1979). The posterior portion of the genioglossus muscle of the tongue contracts to push the tongue body forward and upward; the anterior portion of this muscle also contracts, to stiffen the surface of the tongue and achieve a narrow midsagittal groove.

In the case of most other vowels, a speaker can produce the acoustic effects that would result from a longer SVT by protruding and/or constricting lip opening (Stevens and House, 1955). For example, developmental studies of the speech of young children acquiring American English show that young boys produce lower formant frequency patterns for most of their vowels than girls, though their SVT lengths do not differ. The boys "round," that is, protrude and constrict, their lips. The girls tend to speak with their lips pulled slightly back (Sachs, Lieberman, and Erikson, 1973). The different vowel formant patterns and other acquired acoustic variations signal gender. However, this isn't possible for the vowel [i]. The formant frequency patterns that specify an [i] vowel thus inherently provide a robust SVT-length calibrating signal as well as identifying the sound as an [i]. This was confirmed in a controlled experiment in which adult human subjects were asked to judge a speaker's body size by listening to an isolated vowel. The listeners did best when they heard the vowel [i] (Fitch, 1994). In contrast the fundamental frequency of phonation F0 was not a useful cue for body size, demonstrating that formant frequencies rather than fundamental frequency were the relevent cue.

The Peterson and Barney (1952) perceptual data support this conclusion. When listeners had to identify isolated words that differed with respect to their vowels, without previously adjusting to a particular speaker's voice, their identification of [i]s was almost error-free; only 2 errors occurred in 10,000 trials (Peterson and Barney, 1952). Vowels such as [I], [ae], and [U] were misidentified over 500 times. The only other vowel that had a low error rate was [u], which is in some ways the acoustic mirror image of an [i] (Stevens, 1972). The formant frequencies of a [u] are driven as low as possible, essentially removing most lip-rounding options. The vowels [i] and [u] form two of the "point" or "quantal" vowels that are perceptually most distinct and delimit the vowel "spaces" of all human languages (Stevens, 1972; Carré et al., 1994). The vowel [i], in particular, represents a limiting condition in which the principles of physical acoustics and vocal tract anatomy provide an acoustic signal that best signals the length of a speaker's SVT. As noted above, the muscles of the tongue are drawn maximally upward and forward to produce the anterior constriction of the oral cavity (Fujumura and Kakita, 1977). Cineradiographic data (Beckman et al., 1995), moreover, show that the location of this constriction is limited to the quantal region specified by Stevens (1972).

Nearey's (1979) perceptual data demonstrate the vocal tract "normalizing" value of the vowel [i]; its role in determining the length of a speaker's vocal tract. Nearey's psychoacoustic experiment used computer-synthesized vowel sequences having the form [i]-V-[i]. The initial and final [i]s were in different presentations: the [i]s would be produced by either a short or a long SVT.[2] The middle vowel's formant frequencies varied for each sequence and included the entire range of possible vowels that could be generated by both long and short SVTs. The [i]-V-[i] sequences were generated in a random sequence and presented to listeners who were asked both to identify the vowel and to judge whether it was "natural-sounding." The naturalness was rated along a 10 position scale, from "excellent" to "nonspeech." Both the vowel categories and speech "naturalness" ratings of the middle vowel F1-F2 values varied systematically according to whether the surrounding [i]s specified a short or a long SVT.

The phonetic category effects observed by Nearey (1979) replicated previous experimental data that showed that human listeners interpret speech sounds in terms of their expectations concerning the length of the SVT that produced a particular utterance. Ladefoged and Broadbent (1967) had shown that listeners will identify the same tape-recorded word as an example of *bit, bat,* or *but* when it is preceded by an introductory phrase that would have been produced by a long, mid-length, or short SVT. Nearey's data show that human listeners make these decisions by scaling formant frequencies up or down in accord with an internal model of the supralaryngeal vocal tract.

It would be possible to argue that these effects are analogous to the transpositions that occur when a piece of music is played in another "key." However, Nearey's data on "naturalness" judgments show that human listeners interpret incoming speech signals in terms of an internalized, neurally instantiated model of speech articulation. Acoustic patterns such as that indicated by the symbol "X" in Figure 2-4 that were judged to be extremely

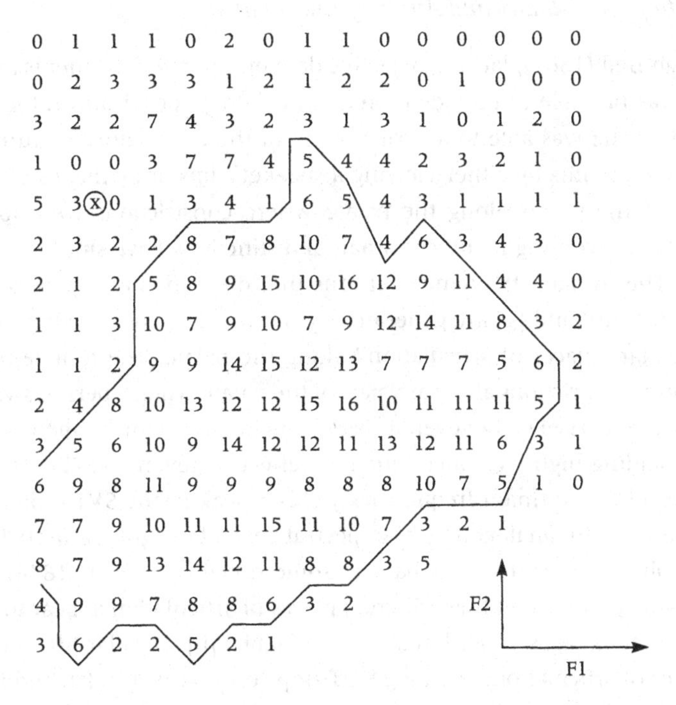

Figure 2-4. The F2-F1 vowel formant frequency combinations synthesized by Nearey (1978) and the "naturalness" judgments made by the listeners who heard these vowels preceded and followed by an [i] having F2-F1 values that corresponded to a long male supralaryngeal vocal tract (SVT). Higher numerical ratings signify vowels that the listeners judged more natural; 10 was a perfect score. The F2-F1 combination at point "X" was judged to be extremely "unnatural"; it fell outside the possible range of a long SVT. This same F2-F1 pattern was within the range of a short SVT; when listeners heard the vowel specified by this same F2-F1 pattern preceded and followed by an [i] corresponding to a short SVT, it was judged to be extremely natural. (After Nearey, 1978.)

good speech signals in the context of short SVT [i]s were judged to be terrible nonspeech signals in the context of long SVT [i]s. Examination of Figure 2-4 shows that the "X" formant frequency pattern could not have been produced by a speaker who had a long SVT. Human listeners, therefore, clearly interpret even vowel sounds by means of a perceptual process that involves articulatory modeling. The studies that follow indicate that the process of internal vocal tract modeling most likely involves the neural substrate that also regulates speech production.

Integrating Articulatory and Auditory Information

Although Bell (1867), lacking objective data on tongue movements and position, was not able to provide correct articulatory specifications for vowel production, he was able to describe many of the articulatory gestures that specify consonants by either viewing a speaker's lips or by means of observations of the points along the palate where constrictions were formed. His claims concerning many consonantal distinctions have since been confirmed. The formant frequency patterns that differentiate stop consonants such as [b], [d], and [g] are generated by momentarily obstructing the SVT at particular "places of articulation" along the palate. The tongue tip and body form constrictions along any part of the palate when a person swallows food (Kramer, 1981). However, at certain points formant frequencies converge, yielding highly distinct "quantal" effects (Stevens, 1872). The convergence of two formant frequencies yields a peak in the SVT's filter function (Fant, 1960), analogous to the spectral peak of a highly saturated color. And as observations that date back to some noted by Müller (1848) show, consonants produced at these discrete places of articulation appear to typify all human languages. English makes use of labial [b], alveolar [d], and velar [g] places of articulation. The long VOT stop consonants [p], [t], and [k] are produced at these same places of articulation and have similar formant transitions. Continuant consonants in which a noise source generated at the constriction formed at the labial and alveolar places of articulation are [f] and [s]. Other places of articulation are used in particular languages; the distribution of sounds may be linked to the relative stability and distinctiveness of the formant patterns generated at a place of articulation (Stevens, 1972).

The perception of the "place-of-articulation" distinctions between consonants likewise appears to involve some sort of implicit knowledge of the formant patterns produced at these discrete places of articulation. One of the effects noted by Liberman and his colleagues (1967) was the "categorical" perception of consonants. They found that although formant patterns that are intermediate between a [d] and a [g] can be synthesized mechanically, human listeners do not "hear" any intermediate sounds when they are asked to identify these sounds; they respond categorically to the synthesized stimuli as either [d]s or [g]s. These articulatory-to-acoustic constraints appear to be structured into the human speech perception system.[3] They reflect the constraints imposed by the human SVT and the principles of physical acoustics (Stevens, 1972; Lieberman, 1984; Lindblom, 1988, 1996). Although "invariant" acoustic cues that are directly tied to the identification of these speech sounds have been proposed (Blumstein and Stevens, 1979), these measures appear to be context dependent for stop consonants (Blumstein and Stevens, 1980), encoded in much the same manner as Liberman et al. (1967) proposed.

The "McGurk" effect perhaps constitutes the most startling evidence that speech perception involves reference to knowledge of speech production and the constraints of the SVT (McGurk and MacDonald, 1976). The effect is apparent when a subject views a motion picture or video of the face of a person saying the sound [ga] while listening to the sound [ba] synchronized to start when the lips of the speaker depicted open. The sound that the listener "hears" is neither [ba] or [ga]. The conflicting visually-conveyed labial place-of-articulation cue and the auditory velar place of articulation cue yield the percept of the intermediate alveolar [da]. The tape-recorded stimulus is immediately heard as a [ba] when the subject doesn't look at the visual display. The McGurk effect can be explained if the speech-mode perceptual system of English-speaking listeners had three categories, [b], [d], and [g], in which they could place the signals that specify these stop consonants. The visual information for [g] with the conflicting acoustic information for [b] would yield identification in the intermediate [d] category. These speech-mode categories need not be innately determined; the neural net modeling study of Seebach et al. (1994) shows that "detectors" sensitive to the formant patterns that specify [b], [d], and [g] can be formed by means of associative learning in a neural net.

Visual information conveying information on the lip gestures used to produce speech is integrated with auditory information in normal-hearing people, enhancing speech intelligibility (Massaro and Cohen, 1995; Driver, 1996). Hearing-impaired people who are trained to "lip-read" often can derive phonetic information that enables them to understand a spoken message. Both hearing-impaired and hearing persons can make good use of the partial specification of speech production available visually (Lindblom, 1996). As Lindblom has noted, it would be difficult to account for these phenomena unless we accept the proposition that the perception of speech involves reference to the articulatory maneuvers that underlie speech and the inherent physiologic constraints of human anatomy. Indeed, speech perception is not a strictly "bottom-up" process in which only primary acoustic or articulatory information is available to a listener. Many studies have demonstrated that what a listener "hears" also depends on lexical and pragmatic information (see Pitt and Samuel, 1995, for a review).

However, some phonetic decisions concerning speech follow directly from the acoustic signal and appear to reflect constraints of the auditory system. Kuhl (1981) has noted that voice-onset time, which differentiates the English stop consonants [b], [d], and [g] from [p], [t], and [k] when they occur in syllable-initial position, appears to be based on auditory sensitivities present in chinchillas and other animals. Moreover, the temporal sensitivity that structures VOT decisions (the 20 msec window that defines the "voiced" English [b], [d], [g] category) also plays a role in localizing sounds and temporal order judgments in human beings (Hirsch and Sherrick, 1961). However, this auditory processing apparently exists in parallel with "speech mode" articulatory-based processing of encoded consonant-vowel (CV) and larger multiple consonant-vowel sequences. Liberman and Mattingley (1985) in their revised version of the motor theory of speech perception note a number of phenomena such as "duplex perception" that would be difficult to account for unless a "speech mode" of perception existed. The speech mode as they envision it implicates a "module" distinct from other aspects of auditory perception. However, the phenomena that they discuss fit just as well within a theoretical framework in which parallel processes, some "auditory," some involving neural articulatory modeling, are implicated in the perception of speech.

Prosody

Speech processing that involves reference to articulatory gestures has also been proposed for prosodic cues (Lieberman, 1967). Virtually all phonetic theories (e.g., Jones, 1932) agree that the melody or prosody of speech has a central linguistic function—segmenting the flow of speech into sentence-like units and highlighting words or phrases by means of "prominence" or "stress." Syntactic analysis inherently operates within the framework of a sentence. The traditional definition of a sentence as a complete unit of thought is in accord with all current linguistic theories.

Again, there is general agreement among most studies that the "intonation" contour that delimits a sentence is determined by the time pattern of the fundamental frequency of phonation (F0). Although some debate persists concerning the time course of the F0 contour that in theory is used to signal the end of declarative sentences in most languages (Lieberman et al., 1984), there is general agreement that yes/no questions in many languages including English end with a rising F0 contour. Independent psychoacoustic data show that the perception of a rising F0 sentence-terminal contour is not keyed directly to the absolute value of the terminal rise. The percept instead appears to reflect a listener's making use of subvocal, neurally implemented, articulatory modeling to derive an inference concerning the laryngeal muscle tensions that existed at the sentence's end.

Independent experimental data show that speakers can place emphasis on a word or group of words by generating a momentary increasing subglottal air pressure and laryngeal tension and by increasing vowel durations (Lieberman, 1967; Ohala, 1970; Atkinson, 1973). These maneuvers result in the "stressed" words having higher F0s and amplitudes than they would otherwise have. When a word is stressed in the early part of a sentence, as, for example, in "Did *Joe* eat his soup?" a momentary pulse in subglottal air pressure is generated in the speaker's lungs and lowers the subsequent alveolar air pressure that would have occurred in the absence of the stress on the word *Joe*. This effect reflects the speaker's programming a complex set of commands to the respiratory muscles that regulate alveolar air pressure over the course of the sentence, without reference to the phonetic details (Lieberman and Lieberman, 1973). Speakers, in essence, appear to plan the length of the sentence that they intend to utter without considering all the phonetic details.[4] During normal conversation speakers generally fill their lungs with more air before they start to utter a long sentence. However, they do not appear to take into account the phonetic details of the words of the sentence. Therefore, sounds such as [h], which result in higher airflows than vowels, reduce lung volume more than low-flow vowels. Alveolar air pressure depends to a great extent on the elastic recoil of the lungs. Higher lung volumes will generate higher alveolar air pressures, all other factors being equal (Bouhuys, 1974). The terminal rising F0 contour of a yes/no question is generated by tensing the lateral crico-arytenoid, vocalis, and crico-thyroid muscles of the larynx (Atkinson, 1973). Since F0 is directly related to the driving alveolar air pressure that activates the vocal cords of the larynx, a lower alveolar air pressure yields a lower F0 for the same terminal laryngeal tension. Experimental data show that listeners do not base their judgment of whether a sentence ends with a terminal rising F0 contour on the absolute value of the terminal rise (Lieberman, 1967). They instead base their judgment on the inferred *articulatory gesture* that generated the F0 contour, taking into account implicit knowledge of speech production.

To summarize, the production and perception of human speech are intimately related. Speech is a very special process that allows humans to transmit information rapidly. The human brain appears to contain neural representations of equivalent articulatory maneuvers that generate the acoustic signals specifying speech sounds. Speech perception likewise appears to involve knowledge of the articulatory maneuvers that can generate the sounds of speech and the constraints imposed by human speech producing anatomy and physiology. However, auditory processes and constraints also play a direct part in determining the acoustic features that human languages use to convey linguistic information.

CHAPTER 3

The Lexicon and Working Memory

This chapter surveys some of the operations that any theory for the neural bases of human language must ultimately explain, as well as the apparent central role of speech in linguistic processes such as lexical retrieval and the comprehension of distinctions in meaning conveyed by syntax through the process of phonetic "rehearsal" in verbal working memory.

Although recent experimental findings have provided valuable insights concerning the possible neural architecture and circuits that support these operations, our current state of knowledge is fragmentary. Moreover, the available data can be interpreted in different ways. In some instances, experimental data that have been interpreted in a modular framework will instead be discussed in light of the distributed architecture of the proposed functional language system. I shall attempt to demonstrate that the FLS theory provides a theoretical framework that will lead to a better understanding of these issues. But as is the case for the relationships that hold between the human brain and other aspects of human behavior, we need to know much more.

The Brain's Dictionary

Linguists and philosophers have been debating the nature of the brain's dictionary for thousands of years. It is clear that the lexicon has a "primitive" evolutionary status. Many animals besides human beings can associate "meanings" with words. However, since humans can produce and comprehend sentences with complex syntax, the human lexicon must code linguistic distinctions such as the argument structure of verbs (whether they are transitive or intransitive, whether they can take direct or indirect objects, etc.), as well as "semantic" knowledge. But it is not clear whether a sharp distinction exists between syntactic knowledge and the real-world attributes of words, such as whether a word is a noun or verb. Theoretical studies such as Croft (1991) suggest that the noun/verb distinction is functional rather than formal, representing the basic dichotomy between objects (animate and inanimate) and actions. Other open questions concern the way in which we access the lexicon: What neural processes are implicated? What information do we access when we attempt to comprehend a sentence? Is syntactic information accessed independently of semantic and pragmatic information?

Recent neurophysiologic and behavioral data challenge linguistic theories that differentiate formal, linguistic "semantic" information coded in the lexicon from real-world knowledge. The neural instantiation of the lexicon appears to be a massively parallel distributed network in which individual words are represented by activity patterns in local circuits along the general principles outlined by Mesulam (1990). These circuits reference the neuroanatomical structures that are involved in the direct perception or execution of the concepts coded in words, as well as the neural circuits that code the phonologic "names" associated with concepts. In other words, the brain's "linguistic" dictionary appears to link circuits that code the concepts referenced in a word to the stored "phonologic" sound pattern that represents the word. The sound pattern of a word, its name, in turn, is the primary key to accessing the semantic and syntactic information that constitutes the meaning of a word. The sound pattern of a word also appears to maintain the word in verbal working memory. Verbal working memory (Baddeley and Hitch, 1974; Baddeley, Thomson, and Buchanan, 1975; Baddeley, 1986; Gathercole and Baddeley, 1993) can be regarded as the neural "computational space" in which the meaning of a sentence is derived, taking account of syntactic, semantic, contextual, and pragmatic information.

Although the data base is sparse and must be extended and replicated, recent experimental data support the claim that linguistic-semantic knowledge coded in the neural lexicon is real-world knowledge. Three studies show that when we think of the concepts coded by a word, we activate the brain mechanisms that instantiate those concepts. For example, the PET data of Martin et al. (1995) show that the primary motor cortex, implicated in manual motor control, is activated when we think of the name of a hand tool. Primary visual cortical areas associated with the perception of shape or color are activated when we think of the name of an animal. Neurologically intact subjects who were asked to name pictures of tools and animals activated the ventral temporal lobes (areas associated with visual perception) and Broca's area. The activation of Broca's area wasn't surprising, since naming deficits occur when low-voltage, current-limited electrical simulation was applied to cortical areas in or near Broca's area in awake patients (Ojemann and Mateer, 1979). The electrical signals applied in Ojemann's experiments block activity in circuits that involve neuronal populations in these cortical sites. Word-finding deficits are common in Broca's aphasia, though as we shall see in the chapters that follow, the linguistic deficits that make up *syndrome* of Broca's aphasia do not necessarily arise from impairment of activity in Broca's area. Moreover, the activation of the primary visual cortex shows that thinking about a word enlists the neural structures that play a part in forming one aspect of the concept coded in the word, the shape or shapes and colors of the object or living being coded by the word. Animal names activated the left medial occipital lobe, a region involved in the earliest stages of visual perception. Moreover, the pattern of activation was not limited to images. The PET data of Martin and his colleagues show that tool names also activated a left premotor area that was also activated by imagined hand movements as well as an area in the left middle temporal gyrus also activated by action words.

A second PET study of neurologically intact subjects who were asked to retrieve information about specific objects and words reinforces the premise that the knowledge "coded" in words is stored and accessed by activating the neuroanatomical structures and circuits that constitute the means by which we attain and/or make use of the knowledge coded by words. Subjects were asked to either name the color associated with an object or word (e.g, "yellow" for a pencil) or state the action associated with the word or object (e.g., "write" for a pencil). As Martin et al. note, "Generation of color words selectively activated a region in the ventral temporal lobe just anterior to the area involved in the perception of color, whereas generation of action words activated a region in the left temporal gyrus just anterior to the area involved in the perception of motion" (1995, p. 102).

It is significant that the areas of the cortex involved in these aspects of visual perception are multisensory. Other neural circuits supported in these regions of the cortex are implicated in tactile sensation and audition (Ungerleider, 1995). Neurophysiologic data again show that Brodmann's area 17, an area of the cortex associated with early stages of visual perception, is activated when human subjects are asked to image simple patterns (Kosslyn et al., 1999).

Studies of "experiments in nature" after brain damage provided the first evidence for the distributed nature of the brain's dictionary. Paradoxically, Caramazza and Hillis (1990) adopt the modular framework proposed by Fodor (1983) to interpret the results of their study of the impaired retrieval of words by aphasic patients. A modular view of language being regulated by brain mechanisms encapsulated from those that regulate other aspects of behavior would argue against the phenomena observed by Caramazza and Hillis. Their study found that verb retrieval was more impaired than noun retrieval in aphasics with left frontoparietal damage, areas associated with motor control. The independent study of Damasio and Tranel (1993) also found language disorders associated with brain damage outside the cortical areas traditionally associated with language. Two of their three patients, who had great difficulty retrieving nouns without any other obvious language impairments, had damage in their left anterior and middle temporal regions. In contrast, the other patient who had a lesion in the left premotor cortex, a cortical area implicated in motor control, had difficulties retrieving verbs. Damasio and Tranel conclude that "the systems that mediate access to concrete nouns are anatomically close to systems that support concepts for concrete entities . . . the systems that mediate access to verbs are located elsewhere and are anatomically close to those that support concepts of motion and relationship in space-time" (1993, p. 4959).

The lexical retrieval studies reported by Damasio et al. (1996) again demonstrate that the neural substrate that constitutes the brain's dictionary extends far beyond the traditional Broca's-Wernicke's area locus. The data suggest that the brain's lexicon is instantiated in circuits that link conceptual knowledge to phonological representations—the sounds of speech. Deficits in naming were studied in 29 patients who had suffered focal brain lesions. The subjects were shown 327 photographs that fell into three general categories: the faces of well-known people, animals, and tools. The subjects were asked to provide the most specific word for each item. The subjects' responses were compared with the responses of normal controls matched for age and education. If their responses matched those of the controls they were scored as correct. If their response did not match they were scored as incorrect *only* when their response indicated that they knew the semantic, real-world attributes of the item presented in the photograph.[1] For example, the response of a person who failed to name the photograph of a skunk was scored as incorrect when the subject's response was "Oh, that animal makes a terrible smell if you get near to it; it is black and white and gets squashed in the road by cars sometimes." The responses of subjects who did not demonstrate that they knew what the photograph represented were omitted from analysis.

Through these procedures, 29 subjects were found who appeared to have intact semantic representations but who couldn't name the photographs. The distribution of naming deficits varied for the subjects: 7 were impaired solely on persons, 2 on persons and animals, 5 only on animals, 5 on animals and tools, 7 only on tools, and 4 on persons, animals, and tools. All of these subjects had cortical and underlying subcortical lesions localized along the temporal pole and inferotemporal regions (all but one had left-hemisphere damage). When the lesions of the subjects were compared with the pattern of errors, the type of error correlated with the location of cortical and subcortical lesions. Naming deficits associated with persons occurred in the temporal pole, those associated with animals in the anterior inferotemporal region, and those associated with tools in the posterior inferotemporal region.[2] Overlapping naming categories were spatially correlated with these regions; for example, the subjects who had naming deficits in all three categories had cortical and subcortical lesions that involved the three cortical subregions. The subjects' lesions "concerned both cortex and subcortical white matter" (Damasio et al., 1996, p. 501).

A PET study with 9 neurologically intact right-handed subjects used a subset of the 327 photographs. The PET data yielded confirming results plus increased activity in the inferior frontal gyrus and anterior cingulate gyrus. Damasio and her colleagues suggest that the localization noted in their study is due to the interaction of the manner in which a person "learns" the meaning of a word and the neural architecture of the cortex. They conclude that

> varied conceptual specification, which results from factors such as physical characteristics and conceptual complexity, is the driving force and "principle" behind the difference in location of the lexical intermediary regions identified here. For example, consider the multiple sensory channels (somatosensory, visual) and the hand motor patterns that are inherent in the conceptual description of a manipulable tool. These would result in the respective intermediary region being recruited near a sector of cortex that is capable of receiving such multiple sensory inputs, and is close to regions involved in visual motion and hand motion processing. (Damasio et al., 1996, p. 504)

Leslie Ungerleider in her 1995 review of brain imaging studies reaches similar conclusions concerning the cortical locus of "knowledge" conveyed by words that refer to objects. She concludes that "information about all the different visual attributes of an object is not stored in a unified fashion in any single area of the cortex. Rather, object knowledge seems to be stored in a distributed cortical system in which information about specific features is stored close to the regions of the cortex that mediate the perception of those features" (p. 770).

Though the data of Damasio and her colleagues do not address the detailed "microstructure," that is, the microcircuits that are instantiated in these intermediary regions, they

> do not envisage them as rigid "modules" or hardwired "centres," because we see their structure being acquired and modified by learning. An individual's learning experience of concepts of a similar kind (such as manipulable tools), and their corresponding words, leads to the recruitment, within the available neural architecture, of a critical set of spatially proximate microcircuits. Thus we expect normal individuals to develop, under similar conditions, a similar type of large-scale architecture, but we also predict ample individual variation of the microcircuitry within each key area. (Damasio et al., 1996, p. 505)

Cortical Plasticity, Sensitive Periods, and Variation

The supposition of Damasio et al. (1996) regarding the phenotypic acquisition of the microcircuits that neurally instantiate words is well founded. Neurophysiological studies indicate beyond reasonable doubt that cortical plasticity is general and extends beyond the bounds of language (e.g., Donoghue, 1995; Karni et al., 1995, 1998; Pascual-Leone et al. 1995; Sanes et al., 1995; Elman et al., 1996; Nudo et al., 1996; Sanes and Donoghue, 1996, 1997, in press; Classen et al., 1998). The particular neural circuits that regulate complex aspects of human and animal behavior are shaped by exposure to an individual's environment within a sensitive period. Neuroanatomical experiments, for example, show that inputs to the visual cortex develop in early life in accordance with visual input; different visual inputs yield different input connections (Hata and Stryker, 1994). In fact cortical regions that normally respond to visual stimuli in cats respond to auditory and tactile stimuli in visually deprived cats. Rauschecker and Korte (1993) monitored single-neuron activity in the anterior ectosylvian visual cortical area of normal cats and cats that had been vision deprived. Neurons in this area in normal cats had purely visual responses. In young cats who had been deprived of vision from birth only a minority of cells in this area responded to visual stimuli; most responded vigorously to auditory and to some extent somatosensory stimuli. Cortical restructuring can also occur in adult primates when sensory inputs or motor experience changes, such as after digit amputation (Merzenich et al., 1984; Merzenich, 1987).

Again, though electrophysiologic and tracer data that map cortical pathways are not available for human beings, imaging and behavioral data indicate that similar processes account for the formation of such basic aspects of vision as depth perception in children. PET data show that both the primary and secondary visual cortex in persons blinded early in life are activated by tactile sensations when they read Braille text (Sadato et al., 1996). Children who have suffered large lesions to the classic "language areas" of the cortex usually recover language abilities that cannot be differentiated from those of other normal children (Bates et al., 1997, 1999). Recent data (discussed in Chapter 4) suggest that plasticity can account for the preservation of language in adult humans after the destruction of cortical areas normally involved in processing language.

Cortical reorganization in response to life's experiences has been demonstrated in fMRI imaging studies. The data of the fMRI study of the human primary motor cortex by Sanes et al. (1995), noted earlier, are consistent with phenotypic reorganization of neuronal circuits as an individual learns to perform new motor tasks. An independent fMRI study of musicians who learned to play stringed instruments at different ages indicates that the cortical representation of tactile stimulation of the digits of their left hands is determined by the age at which they started to learn to play (Elbert et al., 1995). As Elbert and his colleagues note,

> Violinists and other stringed instrument players provide a good model for the study of differential afferent input to the two sides of the human brain. During their practice or performance, the second to fifth digits (D2 to D5) of the left hand are continuously engaged in fingering the strings, a task that involves considerable manual dexterity and stimulation. At the same time the thumb grasps the neck of the instrument and, although not as active as the fingers, engages in relatively frequent shifts of position and pressure. The right hand, which manipulates the bow, participates in a task involving

> individual finger movement and fluctuation in tactile and pressure input. (Ibid., p. 305)

The fMRI imaging data showed that whereas the receptive fields of the digits of the right hand were similar for all subjects, the cortical representation of the digits of the left hands of the musicians was greater than that of non-musicians when the digits were stimulated with light, nonpainful superficial pressure. The number of hours of weekly practice didn't affect the size of the receptive fields. In contrast, receptive fields were larger for the musicians who had started to learn to play their instruments earlier in life.

Similar effects can be noted for the perception of auditory signals in musicians. Magnetic source monitoring of the brains of highly trained musicians showed increased cortical representation for piano tones, but not for pure tones of similar fundamental frequency. The enlargement, which was about 25 percent greater than in control subjects who had never played an instrument, was correlated with the age at which the musicians began to practice (Pantev et al., 1998). Wolf Singer's review (1995) sums up much of the evidence before 1995 for cortical reorganization beyond an early sensitive period outside the domain of language. The critical reviews of Sanes and Donoghue (1994) and Donoghue (1995) are particularly insightful.

In a comprehensive review of neural plasticity and the issue of innateness, Jeffrey Elman and his colleagues (1996) persuasively argue that knowledge of language or other domains is not innately coded in the brain. The general architecture of the network of neural pathways of the brain may, to a degree, be genetically determined, but the microcircuitry that instantiates linguistic knowledge is not. Abundant evidence shows that certain parts of the brain are predisposed to regulate particular behaviors. The left hemisphere of the human brain usually is predisposed to regulate language and handedness. These predispositions may derive from the information that is transmitted to particular regions of the cortex through subcortical pathways. However, other regions of the cortex can subsume this processing after damage to the preferred region. Studies of children who have suffered extensive damage to the left hemisphere cortical regions usually associated with language show that they generally acquire linguistic abilities within the normal range (Bates, Thal, and Janowsky, 1992; Bates et al., 1997; Bates, Vicari, and Trauner, 1999; Elman et al., 1996, pp. 301–317). Clearly, this argues against any detailed innate knowledge of syntax resident in any specific part of the human brain.

A Chomskian "Universal Grammar" that determined the grammars of all human languages necessarily must code the principles that structure grammar in some part or parts of the brain. In principle, the Universal Grammar could be coded in a redundant manner in many parts of the human brain. Redundant, distributed coding of the Universal Grammar would account for the ability of children to acquire language after massive destruction of the neural structures usually associated with language. However, as Elman et al. (1996, pp. 7–16, 357–391) point out, our current knowledge of the mechanisms of molecular genetics indicates that a distributed representation could not be innate; there is insufficient genetic material to code a distributed representation of the Universal Grammar. Given our current knowledge concerning neural plasticity and phenotypic organization of the details of neural circuitry, it is most unlikely a detailed Chomskian Universal Grammar is instantiated in the human brain.[3]

Sign Language

In this light, the shift in modality to gesture that can occur in hearing-impaired individuals who use manual sign language is not surprising. Neuroanatomical structures that otherwise would code the production of speech signals appear instead to code the gestures of complex sign languages (Bellugi, Poizner, and Klima, 1983; Nisimura et al., 1999) in addition to systems that process visuospatial inputs. As Elman et al. (1996, p. 300) note, this is not surprising, since the damaged dorsoparietal and frontal regions of the brain that cause sign-language aphasia are involved in processing visual signals.

Verbal Working Memory

How do we pull words out of the brain's dictionary and "use" them? The mechanism of "working memory" appears to provide a starting point for the solution of this problem. The concept of working memory derives from about 100 years of research on short-term memory. Short-term memory was thought of as a sort of buffer in which information was briefly stored, for example as an intermediate stage in the process of committing it to long-term memory. However, most conceptions of working memory take as its function computation as well as storage. In a series of experiments starting in the 1970s Baddeley and his colleagues (e.g., Baddeley and Hitch, 1974;

Baddeley, Thomson, and Buchanan, 1975; Hitch and Baddeley, 1976; Baddeley, 1986; Gathercole and Baddeley, 1993) showed that a single system, "verbal working memory," was implicated in both the storage of verbal material and the comprehension of sentences. They found that the ability to rapidly comprehend sentences decreased when subjects also had to encode and later recall sequences of digits. A trading relationship existed between storage of verbal material and the processes involved in the comprehension of sentences; both tasks appeared to draw on the same cognitive-brain resources. Baddeley proposed that verbal working memory involves two components: an "articulatory loop" whereby subjects maintain speech sounds in working memory by subvocally rehearsing them, and a "central executive" process.

The data of many experiments (reviewed in Baddeley, 1986; and Gathercole and Baddeley, 1993) show that subjects have more difficulty recalling a series of longer words than a series of shorter words, as might be predicted if the articulatory buffer had a finite capacity. When the presumed articulatory rehearsal mechanism is disrupted by having subjects vocalize extraneous interfering words (e.g., the numbers *one, two, three*) during the recall period, recall dramatically deteriorates. Subjects also have more difficulty recalling phonetically similar words. This effect is independent of articulatory rehearsal and presumably reflects uncertainty induced by similar phonetic "addresses" in the lexicon. Similar effects occur when subjects are asked to recall a sequence of words that are either read or heard. These phenomena have been studied in detail. The effects of suppressing articulatory rehearsal by producing extraneous speech have been replicated many times, even by researchers (e.g., Longoni, Richardson, and Aiello, 1993) who believe that their data refute aspects of Baddeley's theory.[4] The central role that speech plays in the human functional language system is manifested in the "rehearsal" mechanism of verbal working memory whereby words are subvocally maintained using the neuroanatomical structures that regulate speech production. Verbal working memory appears to be an integral component, perhaps the *key* component, of the human functional language system, coupling speech perception, production, semantics, and syntax.

It is clear that biological brains contain different working-memory systems. Recent neurobiological views of these different working-memory systems likewise extend their role beyond storage to include relevant computations. In monkeys, visuospatial working memory has been studied in detail. Visual working memory appears to involve different cortical areas that process "where" and "what" an image is. Goldman-Rakic and her colleagues, for example, found sites in the dorsal prefrontal cortex (Brodmann area 46) that code the location of an object when a monkey first views an image on a computer display, and then must point to it after the image has been blanked out. The ventral prefrontal cortex (Brodmann area 9) appears to code shape and color cues (Goldman-Rakic, 1987). Later studies showed that the different cues were not anatomically segregated, but reaffirmed the existence of visual working memory. Imaging studies (reviewed in Ungerleider, 1995) show that humans likewise have a visual working memory system, which is not surprising given our evolutionary history.

It seems clear that human beings possess a verbal-working-memory system that allows us to comprehend the meaning of a sentence, taking into account the syntactic, semantic information coded in words as well as pragmatic factors. Just and Carpenter (1992) suggest that these different elements contribute to comprehension in a common capacity-limited working memory. The Just and Carpenter model proposes that sentence comprehension involves parallel processing of semantic and syntactic information coded in words as well as such factors as a listener's expectations concerning encountering a verb at some particular point in a sentence, and pragmatic information. Experimental data are consistent with their model and, moreover, show that verbal working-memory capacity differs among individuals. Just and Carpenter first assessed individual differences in verbal working memory by means of the reading-span test (Dahneman and Carpenter, 1980). The task requires a subject to read a set of unrelated sentences such as *When his eyes opened, there was no gleam of triumph, no shade of anger* and *The taxi turned up Michigan Avenue where they had a view of the lake.* After reading these two sentences the subject attempts to recall the last word of each sentence. The reading span is defined as the maximum number of sentences for which a subject can recall the last word for 3 out of 5 trials. Among college students reading span varies from 2 to 5.5 sentences. *High-span* individuals in the Carpenter and Just experiments were those whose reading span was 4 or more, *medium-span* individuals had spans of 3 to 3.5, and *low-span* individuals were those with spans less than 3.

The Just and Carpenter model predicts that syntactically complex sentences should load working memory, since the system is capacity-limited, storing words and meanings as well as carrying out syntactic processing. Experimental data show that this is indeed the case. The recall of end-of-sentence words decreases in the reading-span test when the sentences are more difficult. Final word recall, for example, decreases when sentences like *Citizens divulged that dispatching their first born was a traumatic event to face* are presented instead of the easier sentence *I thought the gift would be a nice surprise, but he thought it was very strange,* which has more common and concrete words as well as simpler syntax. The decrease in final-word recall was most pronounced for subjects who had a low reading span.

The major finding of Just and Carpenter (1992) is that syntactic computations are *not* modular and differ for individuals who have different working-memory capacities for language. This contradicts the claims of Chomskian linguistic theory. Adherents to Chomskian theory such as David Caplan (1987) maintain that the comprehension of syntax is encapsulated; it takes place in a module that considers only "syntactic" information.[5] Moreover, according to Chomsky (1972, 1986), syntactic competence is supposedly similar for all "normal" human beings. Just and Carpenter instead propose that

> people with small working memory capacities for language may not have the capacity to entertain (keep activated and propagate additional information from) nonsyntactic information during the syntactic computations, or at least not to the degree that the nonsyntactic information can influence the syntactic processing. In this view, the syntactic processing of a person with a small working memory capacity is encapsulated only by virtue of a capacity constraint, not an architectural constraint. Individuals with a large working memory capacity may be more able to keep both syntactic and nonsyntactic information activated, and hence their syntactic processing would be more likely to be influenced by the nonsyntactic information. (1992, p. 126)

The strongest support for the modularity of syntax comes from Ferreira and Clifton (1986), who tested subjects on a task in which they could avoid going down a syntactic "garden path" (a diversion) by making immediate use of nonsyntactic information. A person reading the sentence *The defendant examined by the lawyer shocked the jury* could reasonably start down a syntactic "garden path" believing that *defendant* was the subject of the sentence until she or he heard the phrase *by the lawyer.* The animacy of the word *defendant* could lead a reader reasonably to expect that the syntax of the sentence was going to conform to the canonical subject-verb-object form of English, such as *The defendant examined the car,* until the *by* phrase was encountered. At that point the initial "garden path" syntactic parsing would have to be reappraised and abandoned, yielding a longer-than-expected pause on the *by* phrase as the reader recomputed the probable syntactic structure of the sentence fragment. These problems would not occur if the sentence was not a "reduced relative clause" in which the words *who was* had been omitted. The syntax of the full relative clause, *The defendant who was examined by the lawyer shocked the jury,* is evident when *who* is read. Ferreira and Clifton measured reading time as their subjects scanned the words of the reduced relative-clause sentences that had initial animate nouns; they found, as expected, that subjects were constructing a "first-pass" syntactic analysis as they scanned the words of each sentence. The subjects, moreover, spent a long time on the *by* phrase, presumably reappraising the sentence's syntax as they abandoned the inappropriate first-pass, garden-path syntactic analysis and computed the appropriate relative-clause analysis.

In contrast, if subjects did make use of nonsyntactic information to aid their computation of syntactic structure, we would expect readers to avoid the garden path when they appraised the inanimate nature of the word *evidence* in the sentence *The evidence examined by the lawyer shocked the jury.* The readers would realize that the inanimate word *evidence* could not be the subject of a sentence with the verb *examined.* Therefore, they would not be led up the garden-path, subject-verb-X construction on reading the sentence fragment *The evidence examined,* and we would expect a shorter pause when they encountered the *by* phrase. However, Ferreira and Clifton (1986) found that readers spent as much time on the *by* phrase in sentences in which the initial noun was inanimate. The first-pass reading times, determined by eye-tracking data, on the *by* phrases were no shorter when the initial noun was inanimate. The readers therefore did not appear to be taking advantage of the nonsyntactic animate-versus-inanimate semantic distinction, which could, in principle, resolve the syntactic indeterminacy that existed before the readers read the *by* phrase. Clifton and Ferreira concluded that syntactic processing was performed by an encapsulated module that was impermeable to other forms of information.

However, the apparent modularity of syntactic processing observed by Ferreira and Clifton (1986) and taken as a given in many subsequent studies (e.g., Caplan, 1987; Stromswold et al., 1996) appears to result from limited working-memory capacity. Just and Carpenter (1992) performed a similar experiment with 40 high-span (spans of 4.0 and over) and 40 low-span (2.5 or lower) readers. They modified the sentences used by Ferreira and Clifton to be certain that semantic cues showed that the grammatical subjects could not be interpreted as an instrument. In addition, the full-relative version of each sentence was presented using an appropriate, controlled experimental design. Both the low-span and high-span subjects took into account the cues furnished by the relative pronouns, complementizers, and auxiliary verbs in the unreduced relative clause (e.g., *the defendant who was examined . . .* or *The evidence that was examined . . .*). The inanimate initial noun *evidence* of the sentence *The evidence was examined . . .* is another cue for the sentence's appropriate syntactic structure, but only high-span subjects had sufficient working-memory capacity to make use of this information. The same capacity-limited verbal working-memory system appears to activate semantic and syntactic information coded in the lexicon. The syntactic computation is carried out using a "pragmatic" strategy based on animacy. However, only the high-span subjects were able to use nonsyntactic information, whether nouns were inanimate or animate, to aid their comprehension of both the unreduced and reduced relative clauses.

In short, syntactic processing is not modular unless one restricts it to individual subjects. However, as Just and Carpenter note, "modularity was constructed as a hypothesis about a universal functional architecture, a construct that is violated by a finding of individual differences" (1992, p. 128).

Similar effects occurred in the comprehension of center-embedded sentences (*The reporter that the senator attacked admitted the error*) by high-span and low-span subjects. Low-span subjects with reduced working-memory capacities took longer to read complex sentences and had higher error rates than high-span subjects.[6] Low-span subjects had a 36 percent error rate answering true/false questions such as *The senator admitted the error.* The error rate of high-span subjects was 15 percent. High-span subjects were also more likely to maintain two syntactic interpretations than low-span when reading ambiguous sentences such as *The experienced subjects warned about the dangers conducted the midnight raid* (Just and Carpenter, 1992). The effects again appear to derive from individual differences in processing capacity.

These effects would not be surprising if "nativist" linguistic theories were based on biological fact instead of on essentialistic philosophy. As Mayr (1982) notes, variation is *the* feedstock of evolution and characterizes all living organisms. Hence we should expect to find individual differences in linguistic ability that reflect biological endowment as well as phenotypic development.

Several studies that reveal the contributions of biological endowment to personality (e.g., Kagan, 1989) and language have addressed this issue.

Plomin (1989) studied the communicative behavior of identical twins who were raised in different homes during the first year of life. Vocal imitation and the onset of word production were studied. Only 19 percent of the variability in the infants' communicative behavior could be correlated with the cognitive ability of their birth-mothers. In contrast, the correlation between measures of the maternal behavior of the adoptive mothers and the infants' communicative behavior was 0.39. The twin study reported by Dale et al. (1998) found that genetic endowment accounted for only 25 percent of individual differences in language development at age 2 years for a sample of 3000 identical twin pairs raised in different homes. However, biology can affect language development. The behavior of the lowest performing 5 percent of the twins raised in different homes correlated 73 percent, whereas environmental factors accounted for 18 percent of the shared behavior of these language-delayed twins. The message that emerges is that gross differences may have a genetic basis. However, the language development of even identical twins varies. This surely should not be surprising given the fact that brains differ as much as faces, feet, hearts, teeth, and other aspects of anatomy (Ojemann et al., 1989; Ziles et al., 1995; Fink et al., 1997). In fact, Mazziotta's ongoing fMRI studies at UCLA of identical twins show variations in gyral morphology.

Verbal working memory thus can be thought of as the computational space (a loose analogy would be the electronic memory buffer of a computer) in which the meaning of a sentence is derived using semantic, pragmatic, and contextual as well as strictly "syntactic" information. Although some researchers still believe that a specialized "module" carries out the syntactic analysis of a sentence (Caplan and Waters, 1990), this proposal is refuted by the converging evidence of many experimental studies (e.g., Just and Carpenter, 1992; MacDonald, 1994; MacDonald, Perlmutter, and Seidenberg, 1994; Bates et al., 1995; Blackwell and Bates, 1995). Studies monitoring brain activity by means of event-related scalp potentials (ERPs) have been taken as evidence for syntactic processing independent of other situational or linguistic information. Electrical activity is recorded using the techniques of diagnostic electroencephalograms (EEGs) for repeated presentations of a stimulus, for example a tape recording of a sentence that has a potentially ambiguous interpretation. The recordings are then synchronized and averaged to reveal electrical activity associated with the interpretation of the sentence. Certain features of the recorded and processed electrical signals were thought to signify syntactic processing as opposed to semantic or pragmatic information. However, recent ERP studies show that this is not the case (Kutas, 1997). Indeed, subphonetic acoustic differences affect lexical access; speech sounds that are acceptable but that deviate from the prototypical acoustic signal delay lexical access (Andruski, Blumstein, and Burton, 1994). Therefore, we can conclude that human subjects do not compute the syntactic structures of the sentences that they hear or read in an "encapsulated" module of the brain that is functionally and morphologically isolated from other neural structures or circuits.

Grammaticality Judgments

If working-memory capacity is a factor in syntactic processing, overloading the computational "space" should induce agrammaticism. The data of King and Just (1980) show that verbal working-memory capacity limits both verbal recall and on-line syntax processing. Subjects comprehending center-embedded sentences had greater difficulty recalling the final words of these sentences. Linguists, however, often characterize "on-line" sentence comprehension as a "production" effect that does not directly manifest linguistic "knowledge," which they equate with "competence." Grammaticality judgments traditionally are the criteria by which linguists judge the descriptive adequacy of theories of grammar. Thus the "rules" of a linguistic grammar must generate the grammatical sentence *Joe was seen by Susan* and *not* generate the ungrammatical sentence *Joe seen was by Susan,* which has an inadmissible word order, or the ungrammatical sentence *The boys is coming home,* which violates the agreement rules of English. Several studies have shown that aphasic subjects who are unable to comprehend distinctions of meaning conveyed by syntax can nonetheless judge to a reduced degree whether the sentences that they hear or read are grammatical (Linebarger, Schwartz, and Saffran, 1983; Wulfeck 1988; Shankweiler et al., 1989). This finding has led many linguists to conclude that linguistic "competence" is preserved in aphasia; the comprehension deficits are taken to signify an irrelevant "production" effect of little interest to linguistic theory. However, it is unlikely that the neural bases of competence or "knowledge of syntax" are completely independent of "processing" or "production" mechanisms. The grammaticality judgments of aphasic subjects, though above chance guessing, are not as robust as those of normal controls. Thirty percent error rates occurred in the experiments noted above, whereas neurologically intact controls made virtually no errors. The data of Blackwell and Bates (1995) show that similar lapses in grammaticality judgments can be induced in neurologically intact, normal subjects by diminishing working-memory capacity. Blackwell and Bates used a technique similar to that of King and Just (1980). Subjects listened to short sentences while they simultaneously performed a secondary task, keeping a string of numbers in memory. They were asked to listen to a sentence and press a button as soon as they were able to decide whether the sentence was "good" or "bad" while they simultaneously viewed a series of either two, four, or six numbers on a screen. After the complete sentence had been heard and the grammaticality judgment made, the subjects had to view a series of numbers and state whether it was identical with the sequence that they had viewed. Grammaticality judgment errors increased as the number-recall load increased. Neurobiological data confirm that the performance of a dual-task problem will load down the "central executive" component of verbal working memory. The fMRI study of D'Esposito et al. (1995) shows that the cortical locus of the central executive component of working memory, the dorsolateral prefrontal cortex, is activated when subjects engage in dual-task procedures similar to that employed by Blackwell and Bates (1995). Therefore, it is improbable that grammaticality judgments provide direct insight on linguistic competence, independent of the mechanisms by which we comprehend sentences. It is more likely that they derive from the same processes by which we comprehend language. The neurobiological data noted below (Just et al., 1996; Stromswold et al., 1996) support this position.

The Neurobiological Bases of Verbal Working Memory

Evidence from independent PET and fMRI imaging studies of neurologically intact subjects is consistent with Baddeley's (1986) proposal that verbal working memory involves both an "executive" component and the covert "rehearsal" of verbal information—a form of silent speech. These studies show that the neural substrate that supports verbal working memory is a distributed system involving Wernicke's area, Broca's area, other cortical areas, and subcortical structures. Moreover, they show that the neural system that instantiates verbal working memory is dynamic, enlisting additional resources in response to task difficulty. Regions of the frontal lobes of the human neocortex implicated in abstract reasoning and planning (Goldstein, 1948; Mesulam, 1985; Stuss and Benson, 1986; Grafman, 1989; D'Esposito et al., 1995; Just et al., 1996) and other cortical areas are recruited as task difficulty increases (Klein et al., 1994; Just et al., 1996).

PET studies of neurologically intact human subjects confirm a close link between the neural substrates involved in speech motor control and the comprehension of syntax. Stormswold et al. (1996), using PET, studied neurologically intact subjects whose task was to make a grammaticality judgment, a hypothetically "pure" linguistic task (Caplan, 1987).[7] The subject's task was to state whether sentences that differed with respect to syntactic processing complexity and/or the presence of nonwords were "acceptable." Although different schools of linguistic theory hold different views concerning the status of syntax, it is clear that judgments of grammaticality cannot be made unless a person is able to "parse" the sentence's syntax. The study found evidence for increased metabolic activity in Broca's area when subjects read sentences that contained a center-embedded relative clause compared to sentences that contained a right-branching clause. Relative rCBF values reflecting brain activity were obtained by subtracting PET data for center-embedded sentences such as *The juice that the child spilled stained the rug* from similar right-branching sentences such as *The child spilled the juice that stained the rug.* As Stromswold et al. (1996) and many previous studies note, center-embedded sentences appear to be more difficult to comprehend because they place a greater load on working memory. Working-memory load necessarily increases because resolution of the initial noun must be delayed until the intervening clause is processed.

However, syntactic processing cannot proceed without considering lexical information. It is inherently impossible to process a sentence syntactically without first identifying its words and their syntactic constraints, for example the argument structures of verbs (Croft, 1991). And, in fact, a growing body of psycholinguistic research based on interactive-activation models of linguistic representation and processing indicates that sentence processing is lexically driven and takes into account probabilistic, semantic, and syntactic knowledge coded in the lexicon (MacDonald et al., 1994; Bates et al., 1995; Blackwell and Bates, 1995). These data cannot be accessed from the lexicon unless the words of a sentence are maintained in working memory. In this light, a second independent PET study (Awh et al., 1996) is extremely significant.

The data of Awh et al. (1996) show that neurologically intact subjects use neural structures implicated in speech production to subvocally "rehearse" letters of the alphabet, maintaining them in working memory. Subtractions of PET activity showed increased rCBF values in Broca's area (Brodmann area 44) as well as in the premotor cortex (area 6), supplementary motor area, cerebellum, and anterior cingulate gyrus when PET data from a task involving verbal working memory were compared with a task that had a substantially lower working-memory load. These brain regions are all implicated in speech motor control. Electrophysiologic data from nonhuman primates, for example, show that the anterior cingulate gyrus is implicated in regulating phonation (Newman and Maclean, 1982) as well as in attention (Peterson et al., 1988). The left-hemisphere posterior (Wernicke's area) and superior parietal regions also showed greater activity as working-memory load increased. These PET data are consistent with the results of studies of patients who have cortical lesions in these areas: they show deficits in verbal working memory that appear to reflect impairment to phonological knowledge, that is, the sound pattern of words (Warrington, Logue, and Pratt, 1971; Shallice and Butterworth, 1977; Vallar, Betta, and Silveri, 1997).

Therefore, the complementary PET studies of Stromswold et al. (1996) and Awh et al. (1996) demonstrate that neural structures implicated in verbal working memory and in speech motor control are also implicated in syntactic processing. The data show that increased activity occurs in Broca's area when listeners parse the syntactic structures of sentences that have more complex syntactic structures; increased activity also occurs in Broca's area when listeners must simply remember the words of a sentence. The neurobiological data complement the findings of the behavioral studies noted above. They demonstrate that the comprehension of a sentence takes place in verbal working memory, and that speech rehearsal is a component of this process. They also show that activation of Broca's area occurs whether the subject's task is to make a grammaticality judgment or to maintain words in the verbal working-memory system that derives sentence meaning. Broca's area does not appear to constitute a localized "sentence-comprehension" organ as Stromswold et al. (1996) claim. The data of Awh et al, (1996) show that the neural substrate implicated in verbal working memory clearly is not localized in Broca's region; the posterior parietal regions, anterior cingulate gyrus, premotor cortex, and supplementary motor area are all implicated in this process. It is also evident that Broca's area also is implicated in manual motor control (Kimura, 1979). Broca's area and its homologue in monkeys support a functional neural system that generates and monitors grasping and manual gestures (Rizzolatti and Arbib, 1998).

Moreover, the neural system that carries out sentence comprehension is dynamic, recruiting additional resources as task demand increases. The fMRI study of Just et al. (1996) made use of the same "subtraction" technique as Stromswold et al. (1996). Neural metabolic activity was monitored as subjects read sentences that expressed the same concepts and had the same number of words but differed with respect to syntactic complexity. All the sentences had two clauses. The sentences with the simplest syntactic structure were active conjoined sentences (type 1) such as *The reporter attacked the senator and admitted the error.* The same infomation was conveyed by the subject-relative-clause sentence (type 2), *The reporter that attacked the senator admitted the error,* and the object-relative-clause sentence (type 3), *The reporter that the senator attacked admitted the error.* These three sentence types differ with respect to syntactic complexity by several generally accepted measures. Type 2 sentences contain a relative clause that interrupts a main clause, while in type 3 sentences the first noun is both the subject of the main clause and the object of the relative clause. Longer reading times, higher comprehension error rates, and measures of task-related stress occur in type 3 sentences. Fifteen college-age subjects read sets of exemplars of each sentence type while metabolic activity in their brains was monitored by means of fMRI. Measures of comprehension were also obtained as well as mean processing time and error rates. Activity in the left temporal cortex, the superior temporal gyrus and superior temporal sulcus, and sometimes the middle temporal gyrus, Wernicke's area (Brodmann's areas 22, 42, and sometimes 21), increased as the subjects read the sentences with increasing syntactic complexity. Similar increases in activity occurred in the left inferior frontal gyrus, or Broca's area (Brodmann's areas 44 and 45). The processing of the three sentence types resulted in increased metabolic activity as measured by fMRI in areas that were spatially contiguous or proximal to the areas activated while reading simpler sentences. Furthermore, the right-hemisphere homologues of Broca's and Wernicke's areas became activated, though to a lesser degree, as syntactic complexity increased. Moreover, the dorsolateral prefrontal cortex showed bilateral activation for three of the five subjects who were scanned in an appropriate plane (coronal scans). Activation levels in the dorsolateral prefrontal cortex also increased with sentence complexity for these subjects. The dorsolateral prefrontal cortex is implicated in executive control, working memory, tasks requiring planning, deriving abstract criteria, and changing criteria in cognitive tasks (Grafman, 1989; Paulesu et al., 1993; D'Esposito et al., 1995). As we shall see in the next chapter, the dorsolateral prefrontal cortex and subcortical basal ganglia support circuits regulating these aspects of cognitive behavior (Cummings, 1993).

A similar phenomenon was noted by Klein et al. (1994), who compared metabolic activity during word generation in subjects whose first language was English but who were also proficient in French. PET monitoring showed activation in similar areas while the subjects performed tasks in either language. Increased activation in the putamen (a basal ganglia structure) occurred as task demand increased when they were asked to repeat English words in French translation. As the chapters that follow will demonstrate, the subcortical basal ganglia and other subcortical structures play a crucial part in supporting the circuits of the FLS.

In summary, the neural bases of human language are not localized in a specific part of the brain. The brain's dictionary appears to be instantiated by means of a distributed network in which neuroanatomical structures that play a part in the immediate perception of objects and animals as we view them or the gestures associated with tools as we use them are activated. The lexicon appears to connect real-world knowledge with the sound patterns by which we communicate the concepts coded by words. Like other neural structures implicated in language, it is plastic and is shaped by life's experiences. Human beings possess a verbal working-memory system that allows us to comprehend the meaning of a sentence, taking into account the syntactic, semantic information coded in words as well as pragmatic factors. Verbal working memory appears to be instantiated in the human brain by a dynamic distributed network that recruits neural "computational" resources in response to task demands such as syntactic complexity and sentence length. The neural network that is the basis of verbal working memory links activity in posterior temporal regions of the neocortex, including Wernicke's area, with frontal regions such as Broca's area (Brodmann areas 44 and 45), frontal regions adjacent to Broca's area, the premotor cortex (area 6), the motor cortex, the supplementary motor area, the right-hemisphere homologues of Wernicke's and Broca's area, and the prefrontal cortex. The anterior cingulate cortex, the basal ganglia, and other subcortical structures such as the thalamus and cerebellum also are implicated. As the following chapters will show, many of these regions of the brain also play a part in neural systems that regulate primitive aspects of human behavior such as motor control, affect, and emotion.

CHAPTER 4

The Subcortical Basal Ganglia

This chapter discusses the central role of the subcortical basal ganglia in the FLS. The basal ganglia, the structures of our reptilian-amphibian brain, channel sensory information from and to various cortical areas, integrating it with "linguistic" information; they also sequence cognitive/linguistic operations. Because complex circuits link the basal ganglia, thalamus, and cerebellum, the chapter also surveys evidence bearing on the role of the cerebellum and other subcortical structures. However, the focus is on basal ganglia, since their role in regulating speech and language is better attested.

Two sources of evidence are considered. Only human beings possess an FLS that regulates spoken language and complex cognitive behavior. Therefore, it is impossible to employ highly invasive techniques that might reveal the FLS's detailed neural circuitry or the "computations" that are effected in its component neuroanatomical structures. However, human physiology is manifestly similar to that of other, related species, and valid inferences concerning the human brain can be derived from the study of the brains of other species. Therefore, comparative studies that reveal some aspects of basal ganglia circuitry and function will be noted. In some instances, comparable studies of human brains are feasible and will be noted. Comparative studies show that basal ganglia circuits carry out at least three functions:

1. They are involved in learning particular patterns of motor activity that yield a reward.
2. They play a part in sequencing the individual elements that constitute a motor program.
3. They interrupt an ongoing sequence, contingent on external events signaled by sensory inputs.

Neurophysiologic studies show that neural circuits link basal ganglia structures and the cerebellum to prefrontal cortical areas implicated in cognition, as well as to cortical areas associated with motor control. Perhaps cognition consists, as has often been suggested, in internalized perceptual and motor activity. But leaving aside speculation concerning the nature of cognition, neurobiological and behavioral evidence demonstrates that circuits involving the basal ganglia play a part in regulating various aspects of cognition in human beings and other species.

"Experiments in nature" on human subjects constitute the second line of inquiry explored in this chapter. Studies of the behavioral effects of brain damage resulting from trauma or disease provide evidence for the role of subcortical FLS structures. They demonstrate beyond reasonable doubt that subcortical structures are essential components of the FLS. The Broca's-Wernicke's model of the neural bases of language is, at best, incomplete. While language often recovers after humans suffer cortical damage (perhaps reflecting the cortical plasticity noted in previous chapters), damage to subcortical circuits results in permanent language deficits.[1] Speech, lexical access, the comprehension of meaning conveyed by sentences, and various aspects of "higher" cognition are regulated by parallel circuits that involve the basal ganglia and other subcortical structures, as well as neocortical structures. The FLS is a distributed network. Parallel processing occurs in neural structures traditionally associated with motor control, as well as in parts of the brain that have been associated with language, higher cognition, and perception.

Basal Ganglia Anatomy

As the sketch in Figure 4-1 shows, the basal ganglia are located deep in the cerebrum. The caudate nucleus and putamen, which form the striatum, are the principal basal ganglia structures that receive inputs from other parts of the brain. The putamen and caudate nucleus receive sensory and other information from virtually all parts of the cortex and other subcortical structures. In rodents, these striatal structures are not anatomically separated. However, in primates they are distinct and appear to receive inputs from different parts of the cortex. Tracer studies of monkeys show that information from the motor cortex is transmitted by circuits to the putamen, while the prefrontal, temporal, and parietal cortex, as well as the cingulate cortex, send information to the caudate nucleus. Neuronal activity can be observed

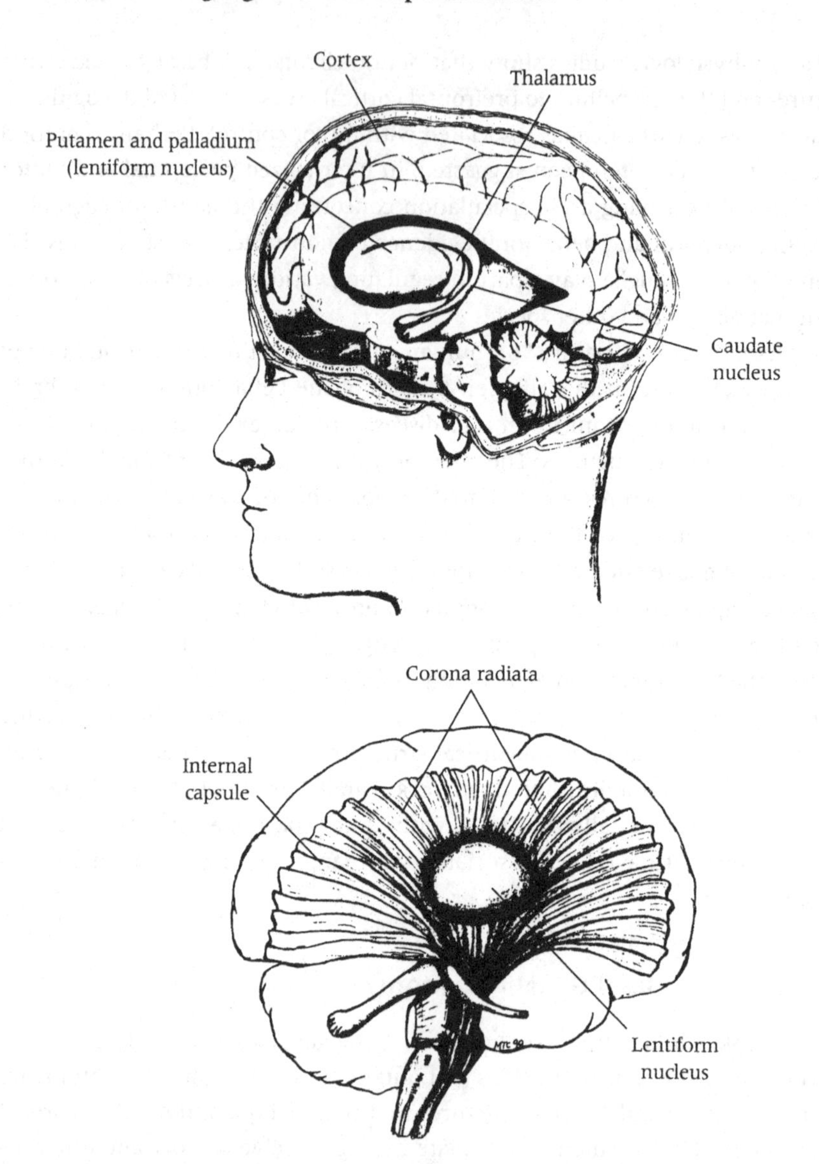

Figure 4-1. The basal ganglia are subcortical structures. The putamen and globus pallidus (palladium) constitute the lentiform nucleus, which is cradled in the nerves descending from the neocortex that converge to form the internal capsule. The caudate nucleus is another primary basal ganglia structure.

in both the putamen and caudate nucleus before movements that are performed by an animal in response to incoming sensory information monitoring the environment (Marsden and Obeso, 1994). Neural circuits also link and transmit information between the putamen and the caudate nucleus (Parent, 1986). In turn, circuits from both the putamen and caudate nucleus transmit information to the globus pallidus (the name "palladium" also refers to the globus pallidus) and substantia nigra.

The globus pallidus, which is often regarded as the principal "output" structure of the basal ganglia (Parent, 1986), has an "internal" segment (GPi) and an "external" segment (GPe), each of which supports segregated circuits to the thalamus, as well as circuits that project back to the putamen and caudate nucleus. Circuits from the thalamus project to various regions of the cortex. Circuits from the basal ganglia also descend to midbrain structures. In mammals at least half of the basal ganglia circuits project to parts of the brain that do not directly initiate motor activity. The complex anatomy of the mammalian basal ganglia constitutes a system that can integrate and process information from one cortical area with other inputs, transmitting its "computations" to other parts of the brain.

One of the major findings of clinical studies over the past decade is that behavioral changes once attributed to frontal lobe cortical dysfunction can be observed in patients having lesions in the subcortical basal ganglia (e.g., Delong, 1983; Delong et al., 1983; Cummings and Benson, 1984; D'Antonia et al., 1985; Alexander et al., 1986; Parent, 1986; Taylor et al., 1986, 1990; Strub, 1989; Cummings, 1993; Malapani et al., 1994). Many syndromes derive from disruption of circuits linking regions of the frontal cortex to basal ganglia structures. Cummings' 1993 review article identifies five parallel basal ganglia circuits of the human brain (p. 873):

> a motor circuit originating in the supplementary motor area, an oculomotor circuit with origins in the frontal eye fields, and three circuits originating in prefrontal cortex (dorsolateral prefrontal cortex, lateral orbital cortex and anterior cingulate cortex). The prototypical structure of all circuits is an origin in the frontal lobes, projection to striatal structures (caudate, putamen, and ventral striatum), connections from striatum to globus pallidus and substantia nigra, projections from these two structures to specific thalamic nuclei, and a final link back to the frontal lobe.

Figure 4-2 illustrates the general architecture of three of these segregated circuits. The motor circuit links neuronal populations in the supplementary motor area, premotor cortex, motor cortex, and somatosensory cortex to the putamen. The neuronal populations in the putamen project to different parts of the globus pallidus. The direct "excitatory" pathway through GPi facilitates movement; the indirect "inhibitory" pathway through GPe provides negative feedback and impedes cortically initiated movements. The circuits from GP are complex; many ultimately project to the thalamus, where outputs to the supplementary motor area, premotor cortex, and motor cortex complete the circuit. Other circuits project directly to multiple cortical areas (Hoover and Strick, 1993; Middleton and Strick, 1994). Reciprocal connections also exist between thalamic nuclei and the putamen and cortex. The dorsolateral prefrontal circuit has a similar complexity, involving connections from Brodmann's areas 9 and 10 to the caudate nucleus and from there through circuits instantiated in neuronal populations in the globus pallidus, substantia nigra, subthalamic nucleus, and thalamus. The dorsolateral prefrontal circuits are anatomically segregated from the motor circuits (Alexander, Delong, and Strick, 1986; Parent, 1986; Cummings, 1993; Marsden and Obeso, 1994). Still other circuits link the basal ganglia, cere-

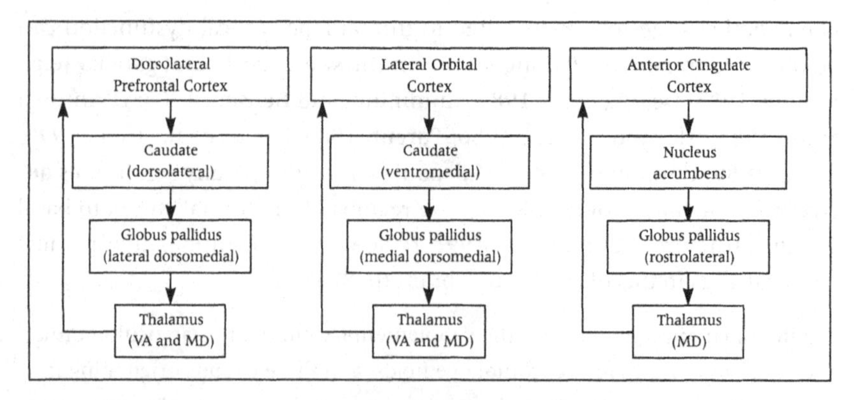

Figure 4-2. Organization of three basal ganglia circuits that regulate various aspects of motor control, cognition, and emotion in human beings. The dorsolateral prefrontal circuit, for example, is implicated in speech motor programming, sentence comprehension, and some aspects of cognition. VA = the ventral anterior region of the thalamus, MD = the medial dorsal region of the thalamus. The diagrams are simplified and do not show the indirect connections of the substantia nigra and other details. Damage to any of the neuroanatomical structures that support the neuronal populations of a circuit can result in similar deficits. (After Cummings, 1993.)

bellum, and prefrontal cortex (Middleton and Strick, 1994). It is apparent that there is as much heterogeneity in the basal ganglia circuits as in the cortex, but we know less about it. We will return to discuss specific aspects of basal ganglia function and circuitry as they pertain to their role in language.

Neurobiological Studies of Basal Ganglia Operations

Syntax of Innate Behavior

To most contemporary linguists the defining characteristic of human linguistic ability is syntax, which allows seemingly infinite linguistic productivity by binding a finite number of words into sentences that can convey an unbounded set of meanings. However, comparative studies of rodents show that they too make use of a "syntax," regulated in the basal ganglia, to bind individual movements into "well-formed grooming programs." The grooming movements of rats do not convey an unbounded set of meanings, or perhaps any meaning, to other rats. They are innate, genetically transmitted patterns coded by a rat "Universal Grooming Grammar" that would be in some ways analogous to the hypothetical Universal Grammar that supposedly structures all human languages. The "forbidden" human experiment, raising a normal child in complete isolation from other humans, can be performed with rats. Rats raised completely isolated from other rats execute these grooming movements, thereby demonstrating that an innate grooming grammar specifies this behavior.

The neural instantiation of this innate rat-grooming grammar can be determined. Experiments performed on rats show that damage to the striatum disrupts the integrity of the *sequences* of gestures that normally occur, but does not disrupt the individual gestures that would make up a grooming sequence. In other words, the "syntax" of grooming is regulated in the striatum (Berridge and Whitshaw, 1992). Damage to other neural structures—the prefrontal cortex, primary or secondary motor cortical areas, or cerebellum—does not affect the grooming sequence. A 1993 study by Aldridge and his colleagues monitored the firing patterns of neurons in the rostral anterior neostratum of 11 rats by means of multiple microelectrodes. Behavior was recorded on videotape and neuronal activity recorded for 23 different behavioral events in sessions that lasted at least 1 hour. The onset and offset times of more than 6,000 events were entered into a computer that correlated frame-by-frame analysis of the grooming sequences with the firing patterns to construct 683 event-time histograms for 31 neurons at 21 recording sites. As Aldridge et al. note (p. 393):

> Sequential syntax of grooming was the main determinant of neuronal responses: Of the neurons that responded to a grooming movement, 85% (29/34) responded differentially to that movement depending on whether that movement was made inside of or within a syntactic chain. At least some neurons responded (with either increased or decreased activity) to each type of grooming movement, although individual neurons showed preferences for particular grooming movements (forelimb strokes vs. body licks). For 47% of the neurons, the sequential context in which a movement occurred determined the neuronal response in an all-or-none. For example, many of these neurons altered their firing during a grooming stroke by the forelimb only when the stroke was emitted within a syntactic chain. When the same stroke was emitted outside the syntactic chain during non-chain grooming, discharge activity was unchanged.

Considering many of the studies of basal ganglia function that are also reviewed here, Aldridge et al. conclude:

> Hierarchal modulation of sequential elements by the neostratum may operate in essentially similar ways for grooming actions and thoughts, but upon very different classes of elements in the two cases . . . Our argument that very different behavioral or mental operations might be sequenced by essentially similar neural processes echoes a suggestion made four decades ago by Lashley (1951). In a paper that defined the issue of action syntax, Lashley noted the continuity between serial order at different levels of psychological complexity, and the continuity this may imply for the underlying neural substrates of syntax. He noted that "language presents in a most striking form the integrative functions [of syntactic coordination by the brain]"; however, "temporal integration is not found exclusively in language; the coordination of leg movements in insects, the song of birds, the control of trotting and pacing in a gaited horse, the rat running the maze, the architect designing a house, and the carpenter sawing a board present a problem of sequences of action [each of which similarly requires syntactic organization]" (p. 113). Circuitry within the neostratum might provide a common sequencing link between phenomena as diverse as actions, words, and thoughts. (1993, p. 393)

Other recent neurobiological studies support Lashley's prescient proposal—that the neural bases of motor control and thought are related. Middleton and Strick (1994) injected a retrograde viral tracer in Walker's (1940) area 46 of the Cebus monkey brain, an area that is known to be implicated in spatial working memory (Goldman-Rakic, 1987; Funahashi, Brule, and Goldman-Rakic, 1993; Courtney et al., 1998) as well as "executive" functions such as planning the order and timing of future behavior (Fuster, 1989; D'Esposito et al., 1995). Clearly, area 46 is *not* a module dedicated to one particular aspect of behavior. The tracer injections did not spread to adjacent cortical sites; they instead labeled neurons in three areas of the thalamus, the dentate nucleus of the cerebellum, and internal segment of the globus pallidus (GPi).[2] The results provided evidence for a distinct pathway from GPi to cortical area 46,

> one in which part of the output of the basal ganglia and cerebellum is directed back to regions of the prefrontal cortex that are known to project to these subcortical structures. This creates the potential for closed loops between the prefrontal cortex and both the basal ganglia and cerebellum. These loops would act in parallel with those serving motor areas of the cerebral cortex but would have a "cognitive" rather than a "motor" function. (Middleton and Strick, 1994, p. 460)

Middleton and Strick conclude that "the cerebellum and basal ganglia should no longer be considered as purely motor structures. Instead, concepts about their function should be broadened to include involvement in cognitive processes such as working memory, rule-based learning, and planning future behavior" (ibid.).

Learned Behavior

Comparative neurobiological studies of nonhuman primates confirm the role of the basal ganglia in learned behavior. Basal ganglia circuits that regulate a learned task appear to be shaped by an associative process. Kimura, Aosaki, and Graybiel (1993) studied the responses of striatal interneurons as monkeys learned a conditioned (associative learning) motor task. At the start of the conditioning process, 10–20 percent of the 201 neurons monitored showed small responses to the sound. After three weeks of conditioning, 60–70 percent responded to the sound. Injection of a dopamine antagonist reduced response to 20 percent.

Independent studies by Graybiel and colleagues (1994) confirm these results. In a series of experiments they employed tracer techniques to map the circuits connecting cortical areas and the basal ganglia and studied the physiology of neuronal response patterns. They found that inputs from cortical sites that represent a particular body part (for example, a hand), in "matrisomes" in the sensory and motor cortex, project to matrisomes in the striatum. Matrisomes are the multiple sites in neural structures at which a particular muscle is activated in concert with other muscles to achieve a particular goal. Graybiel and her colleagues found that even more convergence occurs in the striatum, where "any given matrisome receives overlapping inputs from the same body-part representation in different subareas of the sensorimotor cortex, so that several sorts of information relevant to that body-part converge" (p. 1827).

Injections of anterograde tracer in the motor cortex in a site that represents the foot, projected forward to multiple sites in the putamen. In contrast, injection of retrograde tracers in the globus pallidus that projected back to the putamen showed that dispersed matrisomes in the putamen converge to a small area of GP. As Graybiel et al. (1994) point out, this architecture is similar to the parallel processing systems that may abstract "concepts" through exposure to examples of rule-governed phenomena (Elman et al., 1996).[3] They note "a provocative similarity between this biological architecture and the network architecture proposed . . . for a supervised learning system" (Graybiel et al., 1994, p. 1827). The similarities between the computational architecture of the basal ganglia proposed by Graybiel et al. and a typical distributed neural network that can acquire "abstract" concepts by means of repeated exposure to noisy inputs (Anderson, 1994) is evident in Figures 4-3 and 1-2.

Graybiel et al. (1994) also suggest a mechanism that would account for a striatal role in reward-related learning. They propose that dopamine sensitive "TANs," striatal interneurons (neurons that connect to other neurons within the striatum), respond contingent on reward. Mirenowicz and Schultz (1996) in independent studies confirm the role of reward-based, "appetitive" activation of midbrain dopamine-sensitive neurons in primates. Monkeys learned tasks when they were rewarded with fruit juice. The striatal architecture proposed by Graybiel et al. (1994) could carry out both associative Hebbian learning and supervised learning in a manner similar to current computer-implemented models of distributed neural networks (Anderson, 1995; Elman et al., 1996).

Basal Ganglia Regulation of Sequencing in Humans

Less invasive techniques show that basal ganglia circuits regulate sequential, self-paced, manual motor control tasks in human subjects. Abnormalities in motor sequencing are one of the signs of Parkinson's disease (PD) (Harrington and Haaland, 1991). Cunnington and colleagues (1995) monitored the activity of the supplementary motor area of the cortex in both PD and normal subjects by means of movement-related potentials (MRPs), electrical signals that are emitted before a movement. The subjects pushed buttons with their index fingers in two experimental conditions. In one condition,

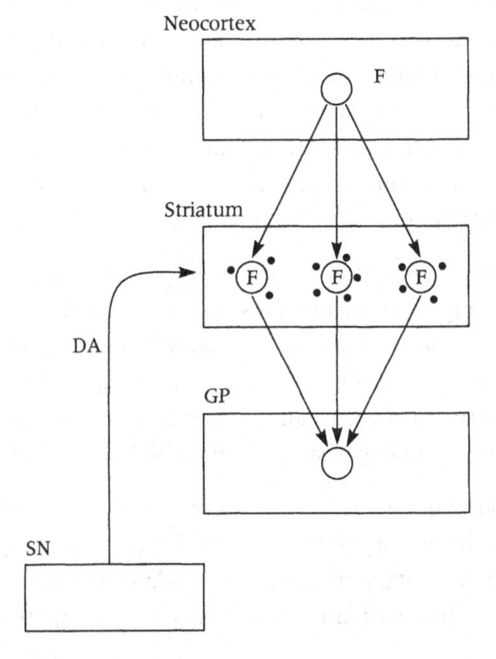

Figure 4-3. The model of divergent-reconvergent computational architecture of the basal ganglia proposed by Graybiel et al. (1994). Experimental data show divergence of inputs from the neocortex to the striatum. A given striatal region can receive inputs from different parts of the sensorimotor cortex. The divergence is followed by reconvergence in the globus pallidus (GP) as well as by inputs from the substantia nigra (SN). (After Graybiel et al., 1994.)

external signals (lights) cued each individual button-push as the subjects pushed a series of buttons that were sequentially illuminated. In the other condition they were asked to push the buttons at an internally generated sequence, for example, sequentially pushing each button of a row of buttons at a five-second interval. Electroencephalogram signals were recorded from the supplementary motor area before and during each button-push. The analysis revealed whether MRPs occurred before the button-pushes, reflecting planning before the execution of these movements. The procedure indirectly monitored basal ganglia activity, since, as Cunnington et al. (1995) note, "The supplementary motor area receives its dominant input from the ventral lateral thalamus, which in turn receives projections almost exclusively from the globus pallidus—the major output unit of the basal ganglia. Consequently, basal ganglia function can be investigated by examining MRPs of supplementary motor area" (p. 936).

The button-pushing tasks executed by normal control and PD subjects in this study included ones in which timing and/or spatial patterns were predictable. Increased premovement MRPs when timing was predictable were present only in normal subjects; premovement MRPs for PD subjects in these conditions were absent or greatly diminished. The data lead Cunnington et al. (1995) to a conclusion similar to that noted by Aldridge and his colleagues for rats, that the basal ganglia

> activate the preparatory phase for the next submovement, thereby switching between components of a motor sequence. Since the basal ganglia and supplementary motor area are more involved in temporal rather than spatial aspects of serial movement, this internal cueing mechanism would coordinate the switch between motor components at the appropriate time, thus controlling the timing of submovement initiation. (Ibid., p. 948)

Studies of spatial sequencing in monkeys support these findings. Sequencing depends on the activity of many cortical areas, including the prefrontal cortex, the supplementary motor area, caudate nucleus, and other basal ganglia structures (Passingham, 1985; Tanji and Shima, 1994; Kermadi and Joseph, 1995).

The difference between the basal ganglia function noted above in rats and primates (including humans) lies in the fact that the manual movements monitored in primates include learned voluntary sequences, whereas the rat grooming pattern investigated was innate. Studies of Parkinson's disease patients consistently show disturbances of sequencing dissimilar learned manual motor movements (Grossman et al., 1991; Harrington and Haaland, 1991), as well as behaviors such as swallowing that are innate (Palmer and Hiiemae, 1998). Similar disturbances in voluntary movement patterns occur for Broca's aphasics (Kimura (1979, 1993) and, as we shall see, may also derive from disruption of basal ganglia circuits.

Stereotaxic Surgery

Since the 1950s, stereotaxic surgical techniques have been perfected that allow basal ganglia structures such as the internal and external segments of the globus pallidus or the targets of circuits from these structures in the thalamus to be selectively destroyed. In the era before Levadopa treatment was available to offset the dopamine depletion that is the immediate cause of Parkinson's disease (Jellinger, 1990), thousands of operations were performed. In many instances these operations reduced the debilitating rigidity and tremor of PD patients. Marsden and Obeso (1994) review the motoric effects of these surgical interventions and similar experimental lesions in monkeys. They address the seeming paradox that surgery that destroys subcortical structures, known to regulate various aspects of motor control, has little effect on motor control though it reduces tremor and rigidity. The answer appears to be, as Marsden and Obeso note, the distributed parallel nature of the basal ganglia system regulating motor control. These findings for human subjects are consistent with neurobiological studies of nonhuman primates. According to Marsden and Obeso,

> With regard to motor processing, it has been found that neurons in supplementary motor area, motor cortex, putamen and pallidum, all exhibit very similar firing characteristics in relation to movement. For example, populations of neurons in each of these regions appear to code for the direction of limb movement (Crutcher and DeLong, 1984; Mitchell et al., 1987; Crutcher and Alexander, 1990), and may alter their discharge in preparation for the next movement . . . Within each of these various motor areas, neuronal populations seem to be active more or less simultaneously, rather than sequentially. They appear to cooperate in an overall distributed system controlling the shape of movement. (1994, p. 886)

The basal ganglia appear to have two different motor control functions in human beings:

> First, their normal routine activity may promote automatic execution of routine movement by facilitating the desired cortically driven movements and suppressing unwanted muscular activity. Secondly, they may be called into play to interrupt or alter such ongoing action in novel circumstances . . . Most of the time they allow and help cortically determined movements to run smoothly. But on occasions, in special contexts, they respond to unusual circumstances to reorder the cortical control of movement. (Ibid., p. 889)

In reviewing the results of many studies that show that basal ganglia circuitry implicated in motor control does not radically differ from that implicated in cognition, Marsden and Obeso conclude that

> the role of the basal ganglia in controlling movement must give insight into their other functions, particularly if thought is mental movement without motion. Perhaps the basal ganglia are an elaborate machine, within the overall frontal lobe distributed system, that allow routine thought and action, but which responds to new circumstances to allow a change in direction of ideas and movement. Loss of basal ganglia contribution, such as in Parkinson's disease, thus would lead to inflexibility of mental and motor response. (Ibid., p. 893)

Experiments in Nature

Only human beings possess language and complex thought, so only data from "experiments in nature" can explicate the role of basal ganglia and other subcortical structures in regulating these singular human qualities. These human studies show that the basal ganglia are essential neuroanatomical components of the functional language system.

Aphasia

The insights gained through the study of aphasia, loss of language from brain damage, have structured theories of mind and brain for more than a century. Aphasiology began with Paul Broca's (1861) study of a patient who had suffered a series of strokes that destroyed an anterior area of the neocortex, "Broca's area" (areas 44 and 45 following Brodmann's 1908, 1909, and 1912 cytoarchitechtonic classifications). The most apparent linguistic deficit of the syndrome named for Broca, "Broca's aphasia," is labored, slow, slurred speech. However, a number of other disruptions to normal behavior that characterize Broca's aphasia have since been noted (Blumstein, 1994, 1995). Deficits in fine manual motor control and oral apraxia typically occur (Stuss and Benson, 1986). Broca's aphasics often have difficulty executing either oral or manual sequential motor sequences (Kimura, 1993). Difficulties in executing sequential speech sounds occur when cortical sites in or near Broca's region are electrically stimulated (Ojemann and Mateer, 1979).

Higher-level linguistic and cognitive deficits also occur in this aphasic syndrome. The utterances produced by Broca's aphasics were traditionally described as "telegraphic." When telegrams were a means of electrical communication, the sender paid by the word. "Unnecessary" words typically were eliminated in telegrams. Hence the utterances of English-speaking aphasics who omitted "grammatical" function words and tense markers producing messages such as *Man sit tree* in place of *The man sat by the tree* had the appearance of telegrams. Aphasic telegraphic utterances were generally thought to be a secondary consequence of the patient's speech motor difficulties; the aphasic speaker presumably was using a compensatory strategy that reduced the utterance's length, thereby minimizing difficulties associated with speech production. The presence of language comprehension deficits in Broca's aphasics that appeared to involve syntax was established by studies starting in the 1970s. Broca's aphasics had difficulty comprehending distinctions in meaning conveyed by syntax (Zurif et al., 1972). Although agrammatic aphasics are able to judge whether sentences are grammatical, albeit with high error rates (Linebarger, Schwartz, and Saffran, 1983; Shankweiler et al., 1986), the comprehension deficits of Broca's aphasics have been replicated in many independent studies (e.g., Baum, 1988, 1989; Blumstein, 1995).[4]

Anomia, word-finding difficulty, can occur in aphasics who have damage to the frontal areas of the cortex described by Paul Broca, as well as in other forms of aphasia. Patients having Broca's syndrome often are unable to name an object or a picture of an object though they appear to be fully aware of its attributes;[5] moreover, they usually have no difficulty classifying words along semantic dimensions. Indeed, Broca's aphasics often rely on semantic knowledge to comprehend the meaning of sentences that have moderately complex syntax. Nonlinguistic deficits also occur; Kurt Goldstein (1948) stressed the cognitive deficits that often occurred in aphasic patients. Goldstein referred to the loss of the "abstract attitude," which resulted in cognitive deficits such as "shifting voluntarily from one aspect of a situation to another . . . keeping in mind simultaneously various aspects of a situation . . . grasping the essential of a given whole . . . abstracting common properties, planning ahead ideationally" (ibid., p. 6). Other studies have reached similar conclusions (Mesulam, 1985; Stuss and Benson, 1986; Fuster, 1989; Grafman, 1989). Despite this constellation of deficits, Broca's aphasia is often characterized as an "expressive" language deficit.

In 1874, shortly after Broca's discovery, Wernicke described different language deficits that hypothetically resulted from damage to a posterior area of the cortex. The most obvious difference between Broca's and Wernicke's aphasia is that the speech of Wernicke's aphasics is fluent. Wernicke's aphasics also have comprehension deficits, and the syndrome is traditionally classified as "receptive." The ability of Wernicke's aphasics to produce and understand language is severely compromised. Though their speech is not distorted, it is often "empty." As Blumstein (1995) notes, the syllabic structure of real words may be altered by sound substitutions (e.g., *poy* for *boy*) and by apparent semantic substitutions (e.g., *girl* for *boy*). In some cases neologisms are produced, nonexistent words that conform to the phonetic constraints of the speaker's language (e.g., *toofbay*). The speech of Wernicke's aphasics is laced with high-frequency words and contentless words such as *thing* and *be*. In addition, though speech is grammatically complex, syntactic phrases are often inappropriately juxtaposed; rampant paragrammatism (substitutions of grammatical morphemes and function words) occurs in highly inflected languages. In short, the productive impairments of posterior aphasia instead appear to reflect "phonological" disorders. The coding or access to the phonologic representations of words appears to be disrupted. This view is consistent with the data of Damasio et al. (1996) concerning the brain's dictionary, discussed in the previous chapter.[6]

Speech Production Deficits

The traditional dichotomy linking anterior cortical brain damage to "expressive" and posterior cortical damage to "receptive" language deficits is misleading. Moreover, as we shall see, in itself damage to the cortex does not result in permanent loss of language. Therefore, Broca's and Wernicke's aphasias are perhaps best regarded as syndromes, characterized by particular signs and symptoms (Blumstein, 1994, 1995). Other aphasic syndromes have been proposed that reflect variations in a constellation of language deficits (Blumstein, 1995), but they are not central to the focus of this discussion, the role of subcortical structures.

The research of the past two decades shows that Broca's aphasics have a characteristic speech-production deficit. First, however, it is useful to note the aspects of speech production that are *not* impaired in Broca's aphasia. Acoustic analyses of speech show that the production of the formant frequency patterns that specify vowels is unimpaired, though there is increased variability (Ryalls, 1981, 1986; Kent and Rosenbek, 1983; Baum et al., 1990). Since formant frequency patterns are determined by the configuration of the supralaryngeal vocal tract (tongue, lips, larynx height), we can conclude that the control of these structures is unimpaired in aphasia. The "encoding" or "melding" of formant frequency patterns which characterizes the production of human speech is likewise preserved in Broca's aphasia. Formant frequency encoding derives from two factors. Inertial "left to right" effects inherently encode formant frequency transitions. For example, to produce the sound [t] the tongue blade must be in contact with the palate (the roof of the mouth). It is impossible for the tongue blade to move away from the palate instantly when a person utters the syllable [ti]. Consequently, the formant frequency pattern gradually changes as the tongue moves from its position at the start of the syllable to its position at the start of the vowel [i]. A similar effect holds for the syllable [tu] except that the consonant "transition" flows into the formant frequency pattern of the vowel [u].

However, inertia cannot account for "anticipatory" coarticulation. Human speakers plan ahead as they talk, anticipating the sounds that will occur. Speakers, for example, "round" their lips (move their lips forward and toward each other) at the start of the syllable [tu], anticipating the vowel [u]. They don't do this when they produce [ti] because the vowel [i] is produced without lip-rounding. It is easy to see this effect if you look into a mirror while uttering the words *tea* and *to*. The time course for anticipatory planning varies from one language to another (Lubker and Gay, 1982) and children learn to produce these encoded articulatory gestures in the first few years of life (Sereno and Lieberman, 1987; Sereno et al., 1987). Acoustic analyses of anticipatory coarticulation in aphasics show that Wernicke's aphasics cannot be differentiated from normal controls (Katz, 1988). Moreover, Broca's aphasics, though they vary in the degree to which anticipatory coarticulation occurs, do not differ markedly from normal controls (Katz et al., 1990a, 1990b).

The primary speech-production deficit of Broca's syndrome is deterioration of sequencing between independent articulators, principally between the larynx and tongue and lips. As was noted in Chapter 2, one of the primary acoustic cues that differentiate stop consonants such as [b] from [p] in the words *bat* and *pat* is VOT, the interval between the "burst" of sound that occurs when a speaker's lips open and the onset of periodic phonation produced by the larynx. The essential point is that the sequence in which laryngeal phonation and the release of the stop consonant occurs must be regulated to within 20 msec. Tongue, lip, or larynx gestures are *not* impaired; no loss of peripheral motor control occurs. Broca's aphasics are unable to maintain control of the sequencing between laryngeal and SVT gestures; their intended [b]s may be heard as [p]s, [t]s as [d]s, and so on (Blumstein et al., 1980; Baum et al., 1990). Control of duration per se is preserved in Broca's aphasics, since the intrinsic duration of vowels is unimpaired (Baum et al., 1990). Sequencing deficits between velar and tongue and lip activity also occur in Broca's aphasics (Baum et al., 1990).

The "phonologic" level, the coding of the sounds that specify the name of a word, appears to be preserved in Broca's aphasics for these same sounds. For example, at the phonologic level the acoustic cues and articulatory gestures that specify a particular stop consonant differ when it occurs in syllable initial position or after a vowel. The speech sound [t], for example, is signaled by a long VOT when it occurs in syllable-initial position. In contrast, after a vowel the acoustic cues for [t] are reduced duration of the vowel that precedes it and increased burst amplitude. Broca's aphasics maintain normal control of these cues although VOT sequencing is disrupted for syllable-initial [t]s. These distinctions are general. The duration of a vowel is always longer before a [b], [d], or [g] than before a [p], [t], or [k]. The fact that Broca's aphasics preserve these durational cues indicates that the phonologic "instruction set" for producing stop consonants is intact. The preservation of these durational cues again indicates that the Broca's VOT deficit derives from the disruption of sequencing rather than from impaired ability to control duration. Instrumental analyses of the speech of Broca's aphasics often reveal waveforms showing irregular phonation (Blumstein, 1994). Speech quality is "dysarthric"; noisy and irregular phonation occurs, reflecting impaired regulation of the muscles of the larynx and alveolar air pressure.

In short, although clinical observations of the speech deficits of Broca's aphasia based on auditory analysis often focus on impaired phonation (e.g.,

Miceli et al., 1983; Nespoulous et al., 1988), a major sign of the syndrome is impaired sequencing between laryngeal activity and lip and tongue gestures. This may reflect impairment of sequencing articulatory gestures that are controlled by different neural circuits. Studies of the vocalizations of monkeys and human speech suggest that the anterior cingulate gyrus (part of the "paleocortex") plays a part in regulating phonation in both humans and nonhuman primates. Lesions in the neural circuits involving the anterior cingulate gyrus extinguish the pattern of laryngeal phonation that marks the primate "isolation cry" (Newman and Maclean, 1982; MacLean and Newman, 1988). Lesions in this circuit can also result in "mutism," the complete absence of phonation in humans (Cummings, 1993). In contrast, independent neocortical areas clearly are implicated in controlling lip and tongue speech maneuvers in human beings. Ojemann and Mateer (1979), for example, show that cortical stimulation disrupts the neural circuits controlling the lip and tongue maneuvers that generate human speech. Neocortical areas do not appear to regulate voluntary vocalizations in nonhuman primates; neither cortical lesions nor stimulation affects their vocalizations (MacLean and Newman, 1988; Sutton and Jurgens, 1988).

Cognitive Deficits

Although aphasia is by definition a "language" disorder, cognitive deficits were noted in early studies. Kurt Goldstein, a leading figure in aphasia research, stressed loss of the "abstract" attitude. Goldstein (1948) described the difficulties that aphasic patients had when planning activities and strategies, shifting strategies, formulating abstract categories, and thinking symbolically. Subsequent research has found that these cognitive deficits are associated with impaired frontal lobe, particularly prefrontal, cortical activity (Mesulam, 1985; Stuss and Benson, 1986; Fuster, 1989; Grafman, 1989). But frontal lobe cognitive deficits do not necessarily result from damage to frontal lobe structures. Studies employing PET and CT scans show that damage either to the prefrontal cortex or to subcortical structures supporting circuits to the prefrontal cortex can yield "frontal lobe" cognitive deficits. Metter et al. (1987, 1989) found that all their Broca's patients had subcortical damage to the internal capsule and parts of the basal ganglia. PET scans showed that these patients had vastly reduced metabolic activity in the left prefrontal cortex and Broca's region. Metter and his colleagues conclude that damage to subcortical circuits to the prefrontal cortex yields the behavioral deficits of Broca's aphasia: "difficulty in motor sequencing (documented for hundreds of patients by Kimura [1993]) and executing motor speech tasks, [and] the presence of language comprehension abnormalities" (1989, p. 31).

The Subcortical Locus of Aphasia

The linkage between subcortical brain damage and the Broca's syndrome noted by Metter et al. (1989) is consistent with data from the studies reviewed in the remainder of this chapter. A paradigm shift focusing on the subcortex as well as the neocortex reflects the continuity of evolution. The human brain did not spring forth *de novo;* the basic subcortical structures found in reptiles (Parent, 1986) and amphibians (Marin, Smeets, and Gonzalez, 1998) survive and play a role in the operations of the human brain (MacLean, 1973). In the context of Broca's time it was reasonable to equate the language deficits of aphasia with damage to the neocortex. Language clearly is one of the "derived" features that differentiate human beings from closely related animals such as chimpanzees. We share many "primitive" characteristics with chimpanzees and other animals. Primitive features are ones shared by divergent species descended from an ancestral species marked by these characteristics. Derived features are ones that differentiate a species from other species that have different evolutionary lineages, though they may share a common ancestor. Since only human beings can talk and human beings have a much larger neocortex than apes (Jerison, 1973), it was reasonable to equate a language deficit, impaired speech production, with neocortical damage. Given the background influence of phrenology, localization of language to a particular area of the neocortex was plausible.

Nonetheless, the role of subcortical brain mechanisms in human linguistic ability has been debated almost from the publication of Broca's studies. Marie (1926), for example, claimed that subcortical lesions were implicated in the deficits of aphasia. This was a reasonable supposition, since the middle cerebral artery is the blood vessel most susceptible to thrombotic or embolic occlusion. The central branches of this artery supply the putamen, caudate nucleus, and globus pallidus. Moreover, one of the central branches of this artery is the thin-walled lenticulostriate artery, which is exceedingly vulnerable to rupture. However, the limitations of postmortem examinations of brain damage effectively ended the debate. Brain imaging techniques that allow the structure and activity of normal and pathologic brains to be monitored reopened the issue. Over the past two decades, it has become apparent that subcortical neural structures are *necessary* elements of a functional human language system. As Stuss and Benson note in their review of studies of aphasia, damage to "the Broca area alone or to its immediate surroundings . . . is insufficient to produce the full syndrome of Broca's aphasia . . . The full, permanent syndrome (big Broca) invariably indicates larger dominant hemisphere destruction . . . deep into the insula and adjacent white matter and possibly including basal ganglia" (1986, p. 161).

A series of independent studies that started in the 1980s show that subcortical damage that leaves Broca's area intact can result in Broca-like speech production deficits (Naeser et al., 1982; Alexander, Naeser, and Palumbo, 1987; Dronkers et al., 1992; Mega and Alexander, 1994). Damage to the internal capsule (the nerve fibers that connect the neocortex to subcortical structures as well as to ascending fibers), the putamen, and the caudate nucleus can yield impaired speech production and agrammatism similar to that of the classic aphasias as well as other cognitive deficits (Naeser et al., 1982; Alexander, Naeser, and Palumbo, 1987). Alexander, Naeser, and Palumbo (1987) reviewed nineteen cases of aphasia with language impairments that ranged from fairly mild disorders in the patient's ability to recall words, to "global aphasia," in which the patient produced very limited "dysarthric" nonpropositional speech and was not able to comprehend syntax. Lesions in the basal ganglia and/or other pathways from the neocortex were noted for all the cases. In general, severe language deficits occurred in patients who had suffered the most extensive subcortical brain damage. The patients also suffered paralysis of their dominant right hands or had difficulty executing fine motor control. Difficulty executing dominant hand maneuvers that require precision and power generally accompanies permanent aphasia (Stuss and Benson, 1986; Kimura, 1993).

Other studies confirm that subcortical brain damage yields similar behavioral deficits (Damasio, 1991; Mega and Alexander, 1994). Patients with stroke damage confined to the basal ganglia have diminished response to rehabilitation efforts (Miyai et al., 1997). It is evident that the neuroanatomical basis of Broca's aphasia is *not* simply a lesion localized to this region of the neocortex. The brain damage traditionally associated with Wernicke's aphasia includes the posterior region of the left temporal gyrus (Wernicke's area) but often extends to the supramarginal and angular gyrus, again with damage to subcortical white matter below (Damasio, 1991). Indeed, recent data indicate that premorbid linguistic capability can be recovered after complete destruction of Wernicke's area (Lieberman et al., in submission). After a stroke in December 1989, sixty-year-old subject, "W," showed the critical features of Wernicke's aphasia, including auditory comprehension deficits and fluently articulated speech containing paraphasic errors; words were produced with inappropriate sounds or syllables, whole-word substitutions, or even neologisms. W was also unable to produce any handwriting and had minor right manual motor control deficits, demonstrating a language- and handedness-dominant left hemisphere. In a 1996 neurological evaluation and a blind evaluation of language performance, W's linguistic behavior showed no signs of Wernicke's aphasia. A comparison of tape recordings of W's speech made before the stroke and in 1996 showed no differences in syntax or phonetic detail. Acoustic analysis showed no VOT sequencing errors and similar formant frequencies, durations, and so on for speech produced before the stroke and that produced seven years later. The comparisons of tape recordings made before and after the stroke show that W retains the speech mannerisms, dialect, lexicon, and syntax that characterized his prestroke speech. Nonetheless, MR imaging performed in May 1993, 41 months after the stroke, showed a left-hemisphere lesion encompassing all of Wernicke's area and adjacent regions of the cortex. The lesion included the supramarginal gyrus; the longitudinal fasciculus was also involved. The data indicate that Wernicke's area does appear to play a part in language; W initially lost linguistic ability after the stroke, consistent with damage to this area. However, the linguistic knowledge or skills that were coded or regulated in Wernicke's area in W's brain must have had distributed, redundant representations, since he did not relearn language.

Thus, in their study of aphasia deriving from subcortical damage, D'Esposito and Alexander (1995) conclude: "That a *purely* cortical lesion—even a macroscopic one—can produce Broca's or Wernicke's aphasia has never been demonstrated" (p. 41).

Neurodegenerative Diseases

Diseases such as Parkinson's disease (PD) and progressive supranuclear palsy (PSP) result in major damage to the subcortical basal ganglia, mostly sparing the cortex until the late stages of these diseases, when cortical receptors may become damaged (Jellinger, 1990). Therefore, studies of the behavioral effects of these diseases can illuminate the role of the basal ganglia in the functional language system. The primary deficits of these diseases are motoric; tremors, rigidity, and repeated movement patterns occur. However, subcortical diseases also cause linguistic and cognitive deficits. In extreme form the deficits associated with these subcortical diseases constitute a dementia (Albert, Feldman, and Willis, 1974; Cummings and Benson, 1984; Xuerob et al., 1990). Deficits in the comprehension of syntax have been noted in several studies of PD (Lieberman et al., 1990, 1992; Grossman et al., 1991, 1993; Natsopoulos et al., 1994; Lieberman and Tseng, in submission; Nakano et al., in preparation; Hochstadt, 1997). A pattern of speech production, syntax, and cognitive deficits similar to those typical of Broca's aphasia can occur in even mild and moderately impaired PD patients (Taylor, Saint-Cyr, and Lang, 1986, 1990; Gotham et al., 1988; Morris et al., 1989; Harrington and Haaland, 1991; Lange et al., 1992; Lieberman et al., 1992).

Dementia has long been associated with Huntington's disease, a neurodegenerative disease that systematically destroys the caudate nucleus but also affects the cortex (Bruyn, 1969). Motor and attentional deficits occur in early stages of the disease and interfere with the normal activities of daily life (Rothlind et al., 1993). Progressive deterioration of sequential motor control occurs in later stages of the disease process (Phillips et al., 1995). The speech produced by patients shows simplified syntax as well as word-finding difficulty (Gordon and Illes, 1987). In advanced stages of the disease, severe speech "dysarthia" (irregular and breathy phonation) occurs. Patients in advanced stages of the disease also have difficulty comprehending complex syntax and naming pictures (Wallesch and Fehrenbach, 1988).

Parkinson's Disease and Syntax

The first study that associated grammatical deficits with Parkinson's disease was reported by Illes et al. (1988); their data showed that deficits were similar to those noted in Huntington's disease. The sentences produced by PD subjects often were short and had simplified syntax. However, Illes and her colleagues attributed these effects to the speakers' compensating for their speech motor production difficulties by producing short sentences. A subsequent study of comprehension deficits of PD (Lieberman, Friedman, and Feldman, 1990) showed that syntax comprehension deficits could occur that could not be attributed to compensatory motor strategies. The comprehension deficits noted clearly were not the result of any compensating strategy, since the motoric component of the subjects' responses both to sentences with complex syntax and high error rates and to sentences with simple syntax and low error rates was identical. The subjects simply had to utter the number (*one, two,* or *three*) that identified a line drawing that best represented the meaning of the sentence that they heard. Deficits in the comprehension of distinctions of meaning conveyed by syntax occurred for long conjoined simple sentences as well as for sentences that had moderately complex syntax. Nine of a sample of forty nondemented PD subjects had these comprehension deficits. Cognitive loss was associated with impaired sentence comprehension. Although the subjects who had sentence comprehension deficits showed no symptoms of dementia of the Alzheimer's type, cognitive decline was apparent to the neurologist who had observed them over a period of time.

The test used to assess the subjects' sentence-comprehension deficits was the Rhode Island Test of Language Structure (RITLS) (Engen and Engen, 1983). The RITLS was originally designed to assess the behavior of hearing-impaired children. Therefore, its vocabulary is simple and can be comprehended by six-year-old hearing children, which argues against the comprehension deficits noted by Lieberman, Friedman, and Feldman (1990) deriving from difficulties with vocabulary. Furthermore, vocabulary and sentence length were controlled for the "complex" sentences, containing two clauses, and for the "simple," one-clause sentences. The vocabulary was also similar for the longer, "expanded" simple sentences (e.g., *The boy is picking apples from the front of the house*) and conjoined simple sentences such as *The boy is riding a bicycle and the girl is walking.* The test battery included sentences having syntactic constructions that are known to place different processing demands on verbal working memory in normal adult subjects (e.g., center-embedded sentences, right-branching sentences, conjunctions, "simple" one-clause declarative sentences, semantically and constrained and semantically unconstrained passives, etc.). Neurologically intact subjects make virtually no errors when they take this test. In contrast, the overall error rate was 30 percent for some of the PD subjects. The PD subjects' comprehension errors typically involved repeated errors on particular syntactic constructions. Therefore, the observed syntax comprehension errors could not be attributed to general cognitive decline or attention deficits. The highest proportion of errors (40 percent) was made on "left-branching" sentences that departed from the canonical pattern of English having the form subject-verb-object (SVO). An example of a left-branching sentence is *Because it was raining, the girl played in the house.* Thirty percent of errors occurred for right-branching sentences with final relative clauses, such as *Mother picked up the baby who is crying.* Twenty-percent error rates also occurred on long, conjoined simple sentences such as *Mother cooked the food and the girl set the table.* This outcome indicates that verbal working-memory load is a factor in sentence comprehension; longer sentences place increased demands on verbal working memory.

Similar error rates for nondemented PD subjects have been found in independent studies (Grossman et al., 1991, 1993; Natsopoulos et al., 1994)[7] and by Pickett et al. (1998) using procedures that monitored either sentence comprehension or judgments of sentence grammaticality. Grossman et al. (1991) also tested PD subjects' ability to copy unfamiliar sequential manual motor movements (a procedure analogous to that used by Kimura [1993], who found deficits in this behavior for Broca's aphasics). The PD subjects studied by Grossman and his colleagues were asked to interpret information presented in sentences in active or passive voices when the questions were posed in passive or active voices. Deficits in comprehension were noted when PD subjects had to sequence between a question posed in a passive voice concerning information presented in an active voice or the reverse. Higher errors, for example, occurred when the subjects heard the sentence *The hawk ate the sparrow* when they were asked "Who was the sparrow eaten by?" than when asked "Who ate the sparrow?" Deficits in sequencing manual motor movements and linguistic sequencing in the sentence-comprehension task were correlated. The correlation between sequencing complex manual motor movements and the cognitive operations implicated in the comprehension of syntax is consistent with Broca's area playing a role in verbal working memory and manual motor control (Rizzolatti and Arbib, 1998) in circuits supported by the basal ganglia (Marsden and Obeso, 1994).

Further similarities between PD and Broca's aphasia were found by Lieberman et al. (1992). Voice-onset-time sequencing deficits similar to those of Broca's syndrome (Blumstein et al., 1980; Baum et al., 1990) occurred in PD subjects who also had sentence-comprehension deficits similar to Broca's syndrome (Blumstein, 1995). Forty Hoehn and Yahr (1967) stage 1 and stage 2–3 PD subjects were studied. The Hoehn and Yahr classification assesses locomotor ability and balance; stage 4 subjects are severely impaired. Acoustic analysis showed a breakdown in 9 subjects' VOT control similar to that which typifies the speech-production deficits of Broca's aphasia. The degree of VOT overlap for the PD speakers was determined using a procedure (Miller et al., 1986) that is weighted toward minimizing overlap deficits. An optimum VOT boundary is calculated by systematically placing a boundary at every point along the continuum of VOT values measured for each subject and determining the number of "voiced" ([b], [d], [g]) and "unvoiced" ([p], [t], [k]) sounds that fall into the wrong category, the VOT value that yields minimal overlap being the optimal boundary. Whereas the overlap for normal controls speaking at the same rate as the PD subjects was 3.6 percent, that of these 9 PD subjects was 18.6 percent. Acoustic analyses showed that the speech of the PD subjects was similar to that of Broca's aphasics in other ways; they produced appropriate formant frequency patterns and preserved the vowel-length distinctions that signal voicing for stop consonants when they occur after vowels. The PD subjects who had VOT overlaps had significantly higher syntax error rates and longer response times on the RITLS than the VOT nonoverlap subjects; moreover, the number of VOT timing errors and the number of syntax errors was highly correlated.[8] Semantic information consistently facilitates sentence comprehension in PD (Lieberman et al., 1989, 1992; Grossman et al., 1991, 1992; Natsopoulos et al., 1994; Hochstadt, 1997; Lieberman and Tseng, in submission; Nakano et al., in preparation) and in Broca's aphasia (Blumstein, 1995). PD subjects, for example, consistently make fewer errors comprehending sentences such as *The box was pushed by the king* than for the similar semantically unconstrained sentence *The fireman was pushed by the cook.*[9]

VOT Deficits: Sequencing or Laryngeal Control?

Impaired laryngeal control, perceptually characterized as hoarse "dysarthric" speech, frequently occurs in Broca's aphasia; low-amplitude speech, "hypophonia," is a sign of PD. Therefore, it would be reasonable to suppose that impaired laryngeal control rather than a deficit in regulating sequencing could cause the VOT deficits noted for some PD patients and Broca's aphasics. Impaired laryngeal control may reflect disruption of the neural circuitry regulating laryngeal control, which in monkeys involves the anterior cingulate gyrus, the supplementary motor cortex, and a dopamine-sensitive ascending pathway through the midbrain tegmentum.

A study of Chinese-speaking PD subjects (Lieberman and Tseng, 1994, in submission) addressed the question of whether laryngeal function or sequencing underlies the VOT deficits noted in PD. The study also tested the hypothesis that degraded basal-ganglia and other dopamine-sensitive neural circuits are implicated in VOT sequencing deficits; VOT overlap was determined before and after subjects took medication that was targeted at enhancing performance of dopamine-sensitive neural circuits. Chinese and many other languages make use of "phonemic tones," controlled variations in the fundamental frequency of phonation (F0), to differentiate words. The syllable [ma], produced with a level F0 contour in Mandarin Chinese, for example, signifies *mother*, whereas it signifies *hemp* when produced with a rising F0 contour. Ten Mandarin- and ten Taiwanese-speaking PD subjects (Hoehn and Yahr stages 2 and 3) read both isolated words and complete sentences in test sessions shortly before and after they took medication that increased dopamine levels. VOT overlaps were determined by procedures similar to those of Lieberman et al. (1992). VOT overlap for PD subjects was significantly greater than that of age-matched normally speaking controls for both the premedication and postmedication test sessions.[10] VOT overlap decreased significantly after medication for half of the PD subjects. This outcome is not surprising, since PD patients often respond somewhat differently to medication (Jellinger, 1990). However, although VOT sequencing was generally disrupted for the PD subjects, acoustic analysis showed that they were always able to generate the controlled F0 patterns that specify Chinese phonemic tones. Since the F0 patterns that specify these phonemic tones are generated by precise laryngeal maneuvers (Tseng, 1981), the data suggest that sequencing deficits are responsible for the observed VOT overlaps.

The preservation of the F0 contours that signal phonemic tones in PD subjects who produce VOT overlaps also suggests that the role of basal ganglia structures in the production of human speech is similar to the sequencing of "submovements" of rodent grooming noted by Aldridge et al. (1993). As noted earlier in this chapter, studies of sequential nonspeech motor activity in PD (Marsden and Obeso, 1994; Cunnington et al., 1995) propose a similar role for human basal ganglia circuits. The VOT overlaps that occur in some PD subjects may therefore reflect degraded sequencing of independent motor commands that constitute the motor "program" for a speech sound. If the human neural circuitry regulating voluntary laryngeal activity during speech production is similar to that of New World monkeys (Newman and Maclean, 1982; Hales and Yudofsky, 1987; MacLean and Newman, 1988), then the locus of VOT sequencing deficits may be the coordination of a laryngeal circuit involving the anterior cingulate gyrus, and independent circuits involving neocortical areas that regulate supralaryngeal vocal tract maneuvers. Significantly, no neocortical areas appear to be implicated in the regulation of nonhuman primate vocalizations (Newman and Maclean, 1982; Hales and Yudofsky, 1987; MacLean and Newman, 1988).[11]

Similar VOT sequencing disruptions characterize the linguistically relevant speech-production deficits of Broca's aphasia (Blumstein et al., 1980; Baum et al., 1990; Blumstein, 1994, 1995). Given the fact that permanent aphasia occurs if and only if subcortical damage occurs, disruption of basal ganglia circuits may be the common basis for this speech deficit of Broca's aphasia and PD. The deficit follows from the facts of anatomy, which are the result of the proximate "logic" of biological evolution (Mayr, 1982). It would be logical to have modular, "compartmentalized" blood supply to various parts of the brain so as to limit the damage resulting from occlusion or rupture. But occlusions of the middle cerebral artery and ruptures of the lenticulostriate artery (one of the central branches of this artery) are the usual causes of permanent aphasia. And the central branches of the middle cerebral artery supply the putamen, caudate nucleus, and globus pallidus.

Focal Subcortical Lesions and Sequencing

Further evidence that the basal ganglia regulate sequencing was found by Pickett et al. (1998) for a woman who had suffered brain damage restricted to profound bilateral damage to the putamen and some damage to the anterior caudate nucleus. Behavioral deficits were found that can be attributed to a breakdown in the subject's ability to sequence the activities necessary for speech production, the comprehension of syntax, and some aspects of cognition. The subject showed impaired sequencing of the articulatory gestures that constitute the speech motor programs of English words. Acoustic analyses showed that the subject's speech was degraded as a result of inappropriate sequencing: inappropriate nasalization, unsynchronized consonantal bursts, and peculiar distributions of VOT sequencing occurred. She was frequently unable to properly sequence intercostal muscle activity regulating alveolar air pressure with upper airway articulation, and thus produced transient changes in amplitude. The subject's speech production errors did not involve timing, since the intrinsic durations of her vowels and consonants were maintained.

The subject had a 14 percent error rate when comprehending distinctions in meaning conveyed by syntax on a sensitive test instrument, the test of "Distinctions in Meaning Conveyed by Syntax" (TMS). Age-matched normal controls made no errors. The subject's syntax-comprehension errors appear to reflect an inability to shift conceptual sequences. For example, high error rates occurred when she responded to probe questions in passive voice concerning information that had been presented in active-voice sentences, or questions in active voice concerning information presented in passive sentences. This severely compromised subject had difficulties comprehending simple sentences in the canonical subject-verb-object form of English as well as in syntactic-semantic processing of embedded clauses, where it is necessary to switch to the analysis of new material at clause boundaries. Cognitive deficits involving sequencing also occurred; she had a 70 percent error rate on the Odd-Man-Out test (Flowers and Robertson, 1985), which involves forming a conceptual category, such as sorting pictures by their shapes and then switching to sorting them by size. Cognitive perseveration occurred when the subject was asked to shift from sorting by shape to size or size to shape; she was unable to shift criteria. In contrast, performance was within normal ranges in tests of lexical access and memory.

MRIs showed that damage to the putamen and the anterior caudate nucleus clearly was the neurological basis for these behavioral deficits. A similar pattern of deficits was noted in the single case study of Robbins et al. (in press); deficits in both visual and verbal working memory tests occurred for a subject having unilateral lesions in the basal ganglia restricted to the left caudate nucleus and putamen. The data of Pickett et al. (1998) bring to mind the conclusion reached by Marsden and Obeso (1994), which is worth repeating, that

> the role of the basal ganglia in controlling movement must give insight into their other functions, particularly if thought is mental movement without motion. Perhaps the basal ganglia are an elaborate machine, within the overall frontal lobe distributed system, that allows routine thought and action, but which responds to new circumstances to allow a change in direction of ideas and movement. Loss of basal ganglia contribution, such as in Parkinson's disease, thus would lead to inflexibility of mental and motor response. (P. 893)

Hypoxia on Mount Everest

Other "experiments in nature" suggest that impaired sequencing stemming from transient damage to the basal ganglia can result in speech-production and sentence-comprehension deficits. The history of the "conquest" of

Mount Everest is marked by disasters brought on by impaired judgment. As climbers ascend, the low oxygen content of the thin air brings on hypoxia. Previous studies have shown that hypoxia on Mount Everest does not impair long-term memory (Nelson and Kanki, 1989; Nelson et al., 1990). However, a study of mountain climbers ascending Mount Everest showed that hypoxia results in co-occurring decrements in the sequencing of stop-consonant VOTs, similar to but not as extreme as in PD, and in the time it takes to comprehend simple English sentences (Lieberman et al., 1994; Lieberman, Kanki, and Protopapas, 1995). Although the climbers also made errors of judgment that fortunately did not result in fatal accidents, they did not manifest the deficits that often occur in PD in nonlinguistic cognitive tests.

The ascent of Mount Everest by the "normal" route starting in Nepal involves establishing and frequenting a series of high camps over a three-month period. A battery of speech, syntax, and cognitive tests similar to those used to assess deficits in PD (Lieberman et al., 1992) was administered to five climbers as they first reached each of these progressively higher camps. Radio links were used between Everest Base Camp (at 5,300 meters altitude) to Camps Two (at 6,300 meters) and Three (at 7,150 meters). Few VOT overlaps were found. However, the VOT ranges of their stop consonants converged. As noted before, the "voiced" consonants of English have short VOTs, and the "unvoiced" consonants have long VOTs. The mean VOT separation width was determined by subtracting the longest "voiced" consonant's VOT from the shortest "unvoiced" consonant's VOT for each "place of articulation" ([b] versus [p], [d] versus [t], [g] versus [k]) and calculating the mean for all of the subjects at each high-altitude camp. The mean VOT separation width of all five climbers decreased from 26.0 to 6.4 msec. The time needed to comprehend spoken English sentences also increased. Response times on the RITLS were 54 percent longer at Camp Three for simple sentences that are readily comprehended by six-year-olds. Sentence response time and VOT decrements were highly correlated.[12]

Hypoxic insult to basal ganglia structures sensitive to oxygen deprivation (Cummings, 1993) is the most likely cause of these speech and syntax deficits. Marked behavioral and cognitive disruptions, similar to those noted for frontal lobe lesions, were noted by Laplane, Baulac, and Widlocher (1984) for eight patients with bilateral globus pallidus lesions resulting from extreme hypoxia. Similar losses were noted by Strub (1989) in a study of a subject having bilateral globus pallidus hemorrhages resulting from exposure to extreme altitude. The Everest results are significant, since the subjects were in peak physical condition; unlike PD patients, who experience locomotor difficulties, the climbers were able to ascend to the summit of Mount Everest. At the elevations at which the climbers were tested, manual motor control and locomotion were not impaired. Since basal ganglia structures also regulate these aspects of behavior, it is apparent that they were lightly stressed. Under these conditions a strong correlation between speech production and the comprehension of syntax was evident, suggesting a close link between the neural mechanisms that regulate these aspects of language. It is possible that sentence comprehension was slowed because impaired basal ganglia sequencing affected phonetic rehearsal in verbal working memory (Baddeley, 1986; Gathercole and Baddeley, 1993).

The climbers made errors in judgment that also may have reflected deterioration of the basal ganglia sequencing function, responding "to new circumstances to allow a change in direction of ideas and movement. Loss of basal ganglia contribution . . . thus would lead to inflexibility of mental and motor response" (Marsden and Obeso, 1994, p. 893). In one instance, the climbing leader (who also showed VOT overlaps at this time) insisted that the group climb from Camp Two to Camp Three as previously scheduled, although a meter of fresh snow had fallen overnight. He did not take into account a danger that should have been apparent to an experienced mountaineer: the severe avalanche danger from the fresh snow covering the steep ice slope between Camps Two and Three. The other expedition members refused to follow his suggestion. In another instance, a climber returning from his successful ascent to Everest's summit stopped at a large crevasse on the Ice Fall, one of the most dangerous parts of the Everest climbing route, where a glacier plunges 300 meters down to Base Camp. The climbing route through the Ice Fall must be continually modified by a Sherpa crew assigned to this task; they must reposition the aluminum ladders lashed together that bridge the crevasses as the river of ice tumbles down. The crevasse in question had been bridged at this point several days before by an aluminum ladder, but the ladder had since been moved 10 meters to the right. Instead of looking for the ladder, the climber continued on the former route, throwing his pack across the crevasse he was about to attempt to jump over, despite his heavy insulated climbing boots shod with crampons (twelve pointed steel spikes). Fortunately he was intercepted by one of the Sherpas who maintained the route. More than 10 percent of the climbers who attempt Everest are not as fortunate; hypoxic cognitive dysfunction and the unforgiving forces of nature make a deadly combination. The disastrous 1995 Everest ascent chronicled in John Krakauer's 1997 book was as much a product of a series of errors in judgment and bizarre decisions as of high winds, subzero temperatures, and blinding snow.

One of the findings of the Everest study has been replicated through use of a hypobaric chamber, in which air pressure can be reduced to simulate the effects of high altitude. Cymerman et al. (1999) recorded and analyzed VOT distinctions in fifteen women who were studied at sea level and after 4 and 39 hours of simulated exposure to 4,300 meters altitude. Each woman read the same list of CV words used in the Lieberman et al. (1994) Everest experiments. The focus of the study was to determine whether deficits in the regulation of VOT would correlate with onset of acute mountain sickness (AMS). A behavioral assessment of AMS was performed twice daily for each subject. Changes in VOT regulation occurred for the subjects who exhibited AMS. No cognitive tests were administered in this experiment.

Slow Speech and Sentence Comprehension

Other studies suggest a link between the rate at which a person speaks and the processing limitations imposed on the phonetic rehearsal mechanism of verbal working memory. Lieberman et al. (1989) tested sentence comprehension for 29 people aged 71 to 93, using the Rhode Island Test of Language Structure (RITLS). Although older subjects as a group tended to have higher error rates, there was no consistent age-related increase in syntactic errors for native speakers of American English. Sentences that had relatively complex syntax or were longer tended to have higher error rates. Vowel duration also was measured for 24 of the subjects. Vowels that had long durations as a result of emphatic stress or prepausal lengthening were excluded; instead the three shortest exemplars of the vowels [i] and [u] were measured. As other studies (Smith, Wasowicz, and Preston, 1986) have found, older speakers tended to have longer vowel durations (the average vowel duration was 331 msec (SD 42 msec) than young adults (200 msec) (Umeda, 1972), but individual differences also overrode this effect. For example, the longest (426 msec) and shortest (278 msec) average vowel durations were produced by 78-year-old subjects. The group of subjects who produced the longest average vowel durations (329 msec, SD 33) had the highest syntactic error rates (16–32 percent errors). The group of subjects who produced the shortest average vowel durations (277 msec, SD 48) made no errors on the sentence comprehension test. The correlation between sentence-comprehension deficits and slow speech suggests that impairment of the phonetic rehearsal mechanisms of verbal working memory may limit the comprehension of syntactically complex or long sentences. Independent developmental studies are consistent with this hypothesis. Developmental studies of the rate at which children speak also show that they do not talk as fast as adults (Smith, 1978) and that memory span increases in children as the number of words that they produce per second increases (Hulme et al., 1984). Therefore, the reduced verbal working memory spans of young children likewise may, in part, derive from slow speech. However, it is difficult to exclude possible reductions in working memory capacity that may reflect other aspects of aging, or for young children increased capacity arising from the maturation of the brain. Further research should resolve these questions.

Cognitive Deficits Associated with Subcortical Damage

As noted earlier, cognitive deficits frequently occur in aphasic patients that are similar to those typical of frontal lobe lesions (Stuss and Benson, 1986). Similar deficits occur in Parkinson's disease as the disease state advances (Cummings and Benson, 1984; Flowers and Robertson, 1985; Beatty et al., 1989; Xuerob et al., 1990; Lange et al., 1992; Cummings, 1993). Although both Alzheimer's dementia and PD tend to occur in older patients, the disease processes that cause PD do not lead to Alzheimer's disease (Jellinger, 1990; Xuerob et al., 1990). Moreover, the cognitive deficits of PD are different from those associated with Alzheimer's dementia; instead they are similar to those associated with frontal lobe damage (Bayles and Tomoeda, 1983; Cummings and Benson, 1984; Flowers and Robertson, 1985; Morris et al., 1988; Lange et al., 1992).

These "frontal-lobe" cognitive deficits are not surprising given the body of evidence for a dorsolateral-prefrontal-striatal circuit in humans (Cummings, 1993) and tracer studies in monkeys showing a direct pathway linking the prefrontal cortex (area 46) and the globus pallidus (Middleton and Strick, 1994). Functional magnetic resonance imaging (fMRI) data confirm the cognitive role of the dorsolateral-prefrontal-striatal circuit in neurologically intact human subjects. Mentzel et al. (1998) studied brain activation using fMRI in thirty-one neurologically intact subjects as they performed a computer version of the Wisconsin Card Sorting Task. The task required subjects as they viewed a series of images to form abstract categories into which they sorted the images. Like the Odd-Man-Out test (Flowers and Robinson, 1985), this test measures the ability to form abstract criteria and the ability to create and shift to new criteria. Bilateral activation was observed in the mesial and dorsolateral prefrontal cortex, including Broca's area (Brodmann areas 44 and 45), Brodmann area 46 (implicated in executive control and working memory), the basal ganglia, and the thalamus. Higher activation occurred in the right hemisphere, perhaps reflecting the use of visual material in the test.

The data of Lange et al. (1992) clearly demonstrate that basal ganglia dysfunction in the dorsolateral-prefrontal-striatal circuit in itself produces cognitive deficits. Lange et al. (1992) compared the error rates and "thinking times" of PD subjects when they were unmedicated and medicated on a computer-implemented version of the "Tower of London" test, which assesses planning usually associated with frontal lobe function. Patients who suffer focal frontal lobe damage have difficulty with this test. The PD subjects saw a computer-generated "target" picture of three colored balls in two hoops. The third hoop was empty. The subjects' task was to move the balls in the two hoops of a second computer-generated image presented below the "target" image and match the target configuration. Figure 4-4 shows a target configuration and the initial condition of the problem. The subjects' task was to copy the ball positions shown in the upper picture. The subjects moved the balls from hoop to hoop using a touch screen. Twelve tests that

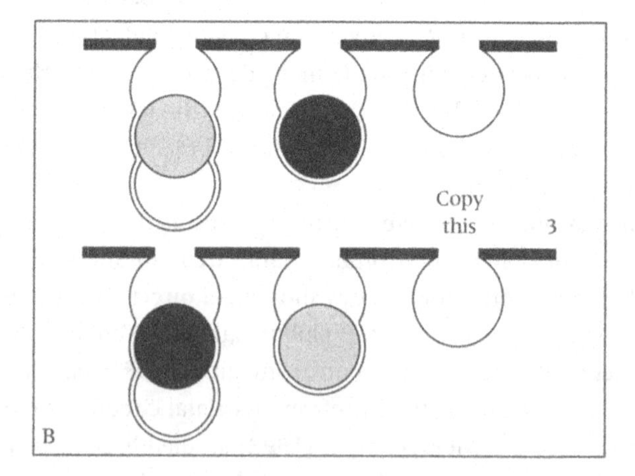

Figure 4-4. The Tower of London test array. Subjects were shown images on a computer equipped with a touch screen and were asked to copy the pattern of balls in hoops shown on the upper part of the display. They could move the balls on the lower display by means of finger movements on the touch screen. (After Lange et al., 1992.)

differed in complexity were presented. The main measure of accuracy of performance was the proportion of problems solved in the minimum number of moves. The time between the presentation of the problem and the first move was recorded as well as the total time needed to solve the problem.

A clever procedure was used to avoid confounding cognitive deficits with the slow motor control that can occur in PD. After each problem a "yoked" trial in which each subject moved the balls following a trace that duplicated his/her movements was used to find the "movement time" involved in each move. Movement time was then subtracted from the execution time of the first move to determine "initial thinking time." The movement time for all the moves was also subtracted from the total problem-solving time. All the subjects had been on levodopa treatment, which restores the level of the neurotransmitter dopamine, thereby ameliorating basal ganglia dysfunction. They were tested when they were medicated and when they had been off medication for several days. Figure 4-5 shows their initial thinking times and the proportion of "perfect" solutions as functions of problem complex-

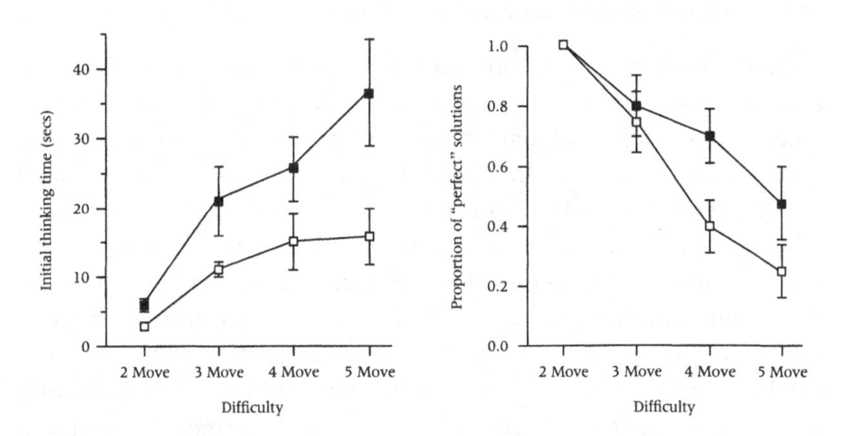

Figure 4-5. Thinking time on the Tower of London test was calculated by subtracting the time that a Parkinson's disease subject took to move his or her finger on command on the touch screen from the time between the presentation of each ball pattern and the same subject's first move. The filled-in squares in A represent thinking time for problems that could be solved in 2, 3, 4, or 5 moves for subjects after they had received L-dopa medication. The open squares plot thinking time in the absence of L-dopa. The number of perfect solutions is plotted in B for the same subjects on and off L-dopa. (After Lange et al., 1992.)

ity, that is, the total number of moves needed for a "perfect" solution "on" and "off" levodopa. Since the subjects served as their own controls, the only factor that differed in the two situations was the activity of the basal ganglia and other dopamine-sensitive neural circuits.

Cognitive deficits also were found for PD subjects by Lieberman et al. (1992). Moderate PD subjects made significantly more errors than mild PD subjects on the Odd-Man-Out test (Flowers and Robinson, 1985), a sorting test that measures two factors: the ability to derive an abstract criterion necessary to solve a problem; and sequencing, the ability to shift to a new criterion. Moderate PD subjects also made significantly more errors than mild PD subjects on other cognitive tests involving working memory—tests of short-term and long-term recall, delayed recognition, and the number-span-backward test—and the Verbal Fluency test, in which a subject must name as many words as possible starting with a particular letter of the alphabet within one minute. Deficits on these tests often occur in PD patients (Parkinson's Study Group, 1989). Performance on these tests was significantly correlated with performance on the RITLS sentence-comprehension test.

Working Memory and Sequencing in Parkinson's Disease

Limits on verbal working memory and cognitive sequencing may interact to cause the language-comprehension deficits observed in PD. The sentence-comprehension deficits of some PD subjects may be due to limits on verbal working memory capacity. In several studies of PD subjects (Lieberman et al., 1992; Hochstadt, 1997; Lieberman and Tseng, in submission; Nakano et al., in preparation), errors in the comprehension of sentences having moderately complex syntax (e.g., center-embedded clauses) or long conjoined simple sentences that also must be held in working memory are twice as high for subjects having VOT overlaps. The data therefore support the view that these errors involve impairment of the phonetic rehearsal mechanisms of verbal working memory. Damage to the neural substrate that regulates speech production (manifested in VOT sequencing deficits) could disrupt the phonetic rehearsal mechanism of verbal working memory. Impaired phonetic rehearsal, in turn, would limit verbal working memory, accounting for sentence-comprehension deficits. However, since similar sentence-comprehension errors also occur in PD subjects who do not have any VOT overlap, disruption of the executive component of verbal working memory (the size of the memory buffer) may also be limiting memory span, yielding sentence-comprehension deficits. Comparative neurophysiologic data show that this is possible. Depletion of dopamine in the prefrontal cortex of monkeys can reduce visual working memory span by affecting the responses of prefrontal dopamine receptors (Brozoski et al., 1979; Williams and Goldman-Rakic, 1997). Therefore, the dopamine depletion that characterizes PD could in itself account for some of the cognitive deficits shared by PD and damage to the prefrontal cortex as well as the sentence-comprehension deficits of PD. Moreover, the transfer of information to prefrontal cortex may be impeded by degraded basal ganglia circuits (Metter et al., 1984).

The data of Pickett et al. (1998) also show that impairment of sequencing in the basal ganglia can result in cognitive inflexibility and consequent deficits in the comprehension of sentences that have embedded or final clauses. The subject also had high errors when she had to answer questions asked in one voice (passive or active) concerning information in sentences presented in the opposite voice, as well as set-shifting in cognitive tests such as the Odd-Man-Out and Wisconsin Card Sorting tests. Similar sentence-comprehension effects were noted for PD subjects by Grossman et al. (1993).

These studies suggest that all of these mechanisms may contribute to the sentence-comprehension errors that can occur in PD. A study that is in progress suggests that limits on sequencing and/or verbal working memory may be responsible in a different degree for the sentence-comprehension deficits of individual PD subjects (Nakano, Hochstadt, and Lieberman, in preparation). In other words, the sentence-comprehension deficits of some PD subjects may be due to limits on verbal working-memory capacity that derive directly from dopamine depletion; other PD subjects may have sequencing problems that affect working memory, cognitive sequencing, or both. Twenty PD subjects having mild to moderate motor impairments were studied. Nakano and her colleagues determined verbal memory span following the procedure used by Daneman and Carpenter (1980). Each subject read a set of sentences and was then asked to recall the last word of each sentence. The number of sentences in each set was increased from two, to three, and to four sentences if the subject had successfully completed the recall task for a lesser number of sentences. Memory span was judged to be higher if the subject could recall the last word of each sentence in a set that contained more sentences. The Odd-Man-Out and TMS sentence-comprehension tests were also administered, and the subjects each read a list of single-syllable words containing stop consonants in initial and final position. Vowel durations, VOTs, and VOT overlap were measured using the procedures of Lieberman et al. (1992). A significantly high correlation was found between reading span and performance on the Odd-Man-Out and TMS tests, except for subjects who had VOT overlaps. In fact the highest error rates on the Odd-Man-Out and TMS tests occurred for the subject who had the highest reading span (3.5 sentences) but whose speech showed VOT overlap and other acoustic events that appeared to reflect impaired sequencing of motor commands. This finding shows that a breakdown in sequencing can result in motor, sentence-comprehension, and cognitive deficits when verbal working-memory span is preserved.

Close examination of the error patterns on the Odd-Man-Out test also showed that other PD subjects who had speech motor sequencing deficits had high error rates when they had to switch criteria on the Odd-Man-Out test, suggesting cognitive inflexibility deriving from an inability to change a cognitive sequence. Still other PD subjects who had both VOT sequencing deficits and sentence-comprehension errors instead were unable to maintain a criterion between trials on the Odd-Man-Out test, consistent with impaired phonetic rehearsal limiting verbal working memory. Similar findings were apparent in a study that tested PD subjects and age-matched neurologically intact controls using the TMS (Hochstadt, 1997). Errors in the comprehension of syntax were highly correlated with errors in cognitive tests such as the Odd-Man-Out and number-span-backward, which tap working memory for both the age-matched controls and the PD subjects who did not have VOT overlap. The PD subjects with speech-production impairment marked by VOT overlap had sentence-comprehension errors that were 80 percent higher than those of subjects with equivalent scores on the Odd-Man-Out test. The implication is that verbal working memory was further degraded in these subjects because of impaired phonetic rehearsal. These results are preliminary and call for further study; what is clear, however, is that sentence-comprehension deficits due to limits on verbal working memory and sequencing occur when basal ganglia circuits are degraded or damaged.

Summarizing, the "experiments in nature" reviewed above demonstrate that deterioration of speech motor control, sentence comprehension, and cognition can result from impairment to the basal ganglia structures. Intact subcortical basal ganglia circuits clearly are *necessary* elements of the FLS. The basal ganglia appear to sequence the elements that compose the coordinated articulatory gestures that generate the sounds of human speech; the basal ganglia also both sequence and interrupt the sequence of cognitive processes involved in the comprehension of distinctions in meaning conveyed by syntax. Since sentence comprehension surely occurs in verbal working memory, impaired speech motor control can also degrade articulatory rehearsal. Therefore, many of the behavioral deficits associated with Parkinson's disease almost certainly derive from impairment of basal ganglia components of circuits regulating sequencing. However, memory span may also be reduced by the dopamine depletion that characterizes Parkinson's disease. The similar, though less extreme, deterioration of VOT sequencing and sentence comprehension in hypoxic subjects most likely derives from impaired globus pallidus function. Damage to basal ganglia control circuits likewise may be the basis of the VOT and some of the language deficits of Broca's aphasia. It also is evident that "nonlinguistic" cognitive processes involve neural circuits supported by basal ganglia structures.

The Cerebellum and Other Subcortical Structures

Most of the cerebellum is a phylogenetically primitive part of the human brain and has traditionally been associated with motor control (Bear, Conners, and Paradiso, 1996). Although the mechanics of the cerebellum's role in motor control are still unclear, recent studies confirm that it "smooths out" and coordinates the action of different muscles (Wickelgren, 1998). The cerebellum also appears to be involved in motor learning (Raymond, Lisberger, and Mauk, 1996). Again, although the processes and circuits are unclear, cerebellar degeneration may result in deficits in "executive" functions generally thought to be regulated by the frontal neocortex (Leiner, Leiner, and Dow, 1991, 1993; Schmahmann, 1991; Fiez et al., 1992; Akshoomoff and Courchesne, 1992; Grafman et al., 1992; Kim, Ugurbil, and Strick, 1994). Planning (Grafman et al., 1992) and the ability to shift selective attention between sensory modalities (Akshoomoff and Courchesene, 1992) are affected. A role in regulating sequential timing in diverse tasks is proposed for the cerebellum by Ivry and Keele (1989). These findings are not unexpected, since tracer studies show circuits linking the basal ganglia, cerebellum, and prefrontal cortex (Middleton and Strick, 1994). In contrast, as in the case of Parkinson's disease, memory is preserved in the presence of cerebellar damage (Appollonio et al., 1993). Further evidence concerning possible linguistic cerebellar as well as anterior cingulate activity comes from PET studies of normal subjects during a noun-verb word-generation task (Peterson and Fiez, 1993). Indeed, Leiner et al. (1991, 1993) propose that the dentate nucleus of the cerebellum, the "neocerebellum," may be adapted for cognitive rather than motor functions. However, it is difficult to interpret the data of the noun-verb association task that has been used in some studies of cerebellar linguistic activity. This task conflates knowledge of English morphology, the process by which nouns can be "turned" into verbs, and semantic association.

A recent study by Pickett (1998) of seven subjects who had damage to the cerebellum shows that its role in regulating speech production and in sentence comprehension and cognition may follow from its links to the basal ganglia. Pickett analyzed VOT speech-production errors and tested sentence comprehension and some aspects of cognition using the test battery used in previous studies of PD, hypoxia (Lieberman et al., 1992, 1994; Lieberman, Kanki, and Protopapas, 1995) and focal basal ganglia damage (Pickett et al., 1998). The tests included the Odd-Man-Out test, Verbal Fluency, and number-span-backward. The data are consistent with other studies that suggest a cerebellar role in cognition and language, but are inconclusive regarding the role of the dentate nucleus. One subject who had suffered damage to the left hemisphere of the cerebellum, with almost complete destruction of the dentate, showed high error rates on the TMS test of sentence comprehension. This subject also showed complete inability to shift cognitive sets on the Odd-Man-Out test. He showed no VOT sequencing deficits. However, a second subject who had suffered complete destruction of the dentate had virtually no errors on the TMS test, scoring better than an age-matched neurologically intact control group. The one subject who had extremely high error rates comprehending distinctions in meaning conveyed by syntax suffered pancerebellar atrophy. He also had high VOT overlap in speech production. He showed no deficits in the cognitive tests. However, it is not possible to attribute the deficits of this subject entirely to cerebellar damage, since atrophy may have damaged pathways to the basal ganglia and other neural structures.

Pickett's (1998) most intriguing finding is a significant correlation (−.64, $p < 0.008$) between the "minimal VOT distance" and sentence comprehension when the scores and speech production of both the cerebellar and normal control groups were collapsed. No correlation occurred between minimal VOT distance and any of the cognitive tests. These correlations are similar to those noted for hypoxia (Lieberman et al., 1994; Lieberman, Kanki, and Protopapas, 1995) and again suggest that sequencing in speech production and sentence comprehension are regulated by a common neural system, the FLS.

Concluding Comments

The focus of this chapter on the subcortical basal ganglia should not be interpreted as a claim that syntax resides in the basal ganglia. As many studies have demonstrated (summarized in Mesulam, 1990), neocortical areas support the neuronal populations that form the distributed networks regulating various aspects of motor control, cognition, and language. Both cortical and subcortical structures play a part in regulating aspects of motor control and cognition outside the domain of language, as noted by Alexander et al. (1986), Grafman (1989), Cummings (1993), DeLong (1993), and others. Neocortical areas traditionally associated with language, Broca's area (Brodmann areas 44 and 45), Wernicke's area, and adjacent regions of the neocortex (e.g., Brodmann area 46) implicated in working memory and executive control are implicated in the FLS (e.g., Ojemann and Mateer, 1979; Kimura, 1993; Klein et al., 1994; D'Esposito et al., 1996; Just et al., 1996; Mentzel et al., 1998), as well as the premotor cortex, supplementary motor area, and areas of the posterior cortex (Martin et al., 1995a, 1995b; Damasio et al., 1996) that have been associated with perception and phonologic association. Other subcortical structures that have not been discussed in detail, such as the anterior cingulate gyrus, are implicated in the FLS; lesions in this structure as well as in the supplementary motor area can result in mutism (Cummings, 1993). In short, the circuits of the FLS, like other functional neural systems, involve many neuroanatomical structures, many of which also play a part in regulating other aspects of behavior (Mesulam, 1985, 1990).

However, the experiments in nature that have been discussed demonstrate that subcortical circuits are key elements of the human functional language system. Neurobiological studies reveal the nature of some of the computations performed in the basal ganglia and suggest that segregated circuits instantiated in the putamen, caudate nucleus, globus pallidus, substantia nigra, thalamus, subthalamic nucleus, cerebellum, and anterior cingulate gyrus form part of the FLS. The variable nature of the deficits, induced by strokes and trauma, that can occur in individual cases of aphasia most likely derives from damage limited to particular, anatomically segregated circuits. A localized lesion could disrupt some but not all of the circuits. The progressive course of symptoms that often occurs in Parkinson's disease also probably derives from the segregated nature of these circuits. Tremor, rigidity, and locomotor deficits usually occur first. These motor problems undoubtedly reflect dopamine depletion initially affecting the putamen, which appears to support many motor control circuits. As the disease state advances, the caudate nucleus and other basal ganglia structures supporting circuits that project to prefrontal regions implicated in cognition are affected (Delong, 1993; Parent, 1983).

Sequencing is one of the key operations performed in the basal ganglia and perhaps the cerebellum. Damage to anatomically close but segregated circuits that regulate speech motor activity through projections to the premotor and motor cortex, and syntax through projections to the prefrontal cortex (Brodmann areas 45 and 46 in all likelihood)[13] appears to produce highly correlated sequencing deficits that result in VOT overlap, errors in comprehension of syntax, and cognitive rigidity. The anatomical proximity of these circuits perhaps reflects the evolutionary history of the human FLS (a possibility discussed in the next chapter). Moreover, direct anatomical links between the circuits regulating sequencing of speech motor commands and syntax also may exist. Anatomical evidence raises the possibility that basal ganglia microcircuits may be anatomically linked. Percheron, Yelnick, and Francois (1984) found extensive dendritic arborization connecting neurons in some of the output structures of the basal ganglia (medial globus pallidus and substantia nigra pars reticula). The dendrite tree of only a few neurons in these areas is sufficient to connect to all the neurons of these structures. These anatomical interconnections have led Percheron and his colleagues to conclude that these neurons might transmit information "from different parts of the body" and might "integrate 'motor,' 'oculomotor,' 'limbic,' and two types of 'prefrontal' signals according to context" (Percheron and Fillon, 1991, p. 58).

It is also difficult to separate the effects of impaired rehearsal in Parkinson's disease from the possible effects of dopamine depletion on the central executive component of working memory. Working memory span is reduced when dopamine supplies to prefrontal cortex are depleted. Recent data suggest that both mechanisms, degraded rehearsal and memory span, can result in syntax-comprehension and cognitive deficits in PD (Hochstadt, 1997; Nakano, Hochstadt, and Lieberman, in preparation). Parallel, segregated basal ganglia circuits that play a part in regulating other aspects of cognition (Alexander et al., 1986; Cummings, 1993) may also be degraded in

PD. The progressive impairment of sequencing noted in mild hypoxia, PD, Broca's aphasia, and instances of massive bilateral damage to the putamen may reflect stages of disrupted basal ganglia function. However, basal ganglia impairment of speech motor sequencing may directly account for some of the observed correlations between VOT overlaps and convergence and deficits in the comprehension of distinctions in meaning conveyed by syntax. The data of Pickett et al. (1998) indicate that impaired basal ganglia sequencing can result in degraded speech, sentence comprehension, and the ability to shift cognitive behavior. Moreover, as noted in Chapter 3, the data of many independent studies indicate that subvocal, phonetic rehearsal maintains the words of a sentence in verbal working memory. The PET study of Awh et al. (1996) shows that the neural substrate that is activated when speech is produced is also activated during silent phonetic rehearsal. Therefore, degraded activity or lesions that damage the neural circuits that regulate speech production would impair phonetic rehearsal, thereby interfering with the comprehension of syntax. The data of the Mount Everest hypoxia study, in which locomotor and manual activity obviously was preserved, suggest that a close link exists between impaired speech motor sequencing and the comprehension of syntax in verbal working memory. A similar correlation was noted by Pickett (1998) for cerebellar damage. Other evidence, discussed in the next chapter, such as the absence of speech and syntactic ability in apes and a genetic defect that causes speech and syntax deficits in humans, also points to a close link between circuits regulating sequencing in speech and syntax.[14]

In short, it is apparent that our reptile brain plays a part in language and thought. Subcortical circuits involving basal ganglia are key elements of the human brain's functional language system, regulating speech, comprehension of syntax, and certain aspects of cognition.[15]

CHAPTER 5

The Evolution of the Functional Language System

Since we cannot observe prehistoric people or events, inferences concerning the behavior and physiology of extinct species must be based on evidence drawn from the present. Comparative studies of living species and the fossil and archaeological records constitute our window on the evolution of human language. When one or more living species share "primitive" features, characteristics that appear to have been present in a common ancestor, we can derive reasonable inferences concerning the behavior, anatomy, and brains of ancestral species that are long extinct and reasonable guesses concerning the evolution of "derived" features that differentiate a living species from its ancestral species.

The comparative method has yielded insights on the evolution of human derived characteristics such as walking—upright bipedal locomotion. It is clear that living chimpanzees and humans share many primitive features that derive from a common hominoid ancestral species that lived about 5 million years ago. We share virtually all our genes with chimpanzees (Sarich, 1974). Indeed, the anatomical similarity between chimpanzees and human beings was evident in the seventeenth century (Perrault, 1676; Tyson, 1699). Observations of present-day chimpanzees show that they and we have many things in common: maternal care, toolmaking ability, territoriality, hunting, and warfare (Goodall, 1986). Chimpanzees and we share anatomical and neural capacities that allow these patterns of behavior to emerge in appropriate environments, and so we can be reasonably certain that they are "primitive" and were present in our common hominoid ancestor. Other aspects of behavior, such as erect, fully bipedal locomotion, absent in living chimpanzees, reflect derived aspects of hominid anatomy. However, the evolution of upright bipedal locomotion can be studied because studies of the biomechanics of human walking have revealed the skeletal anatomy necessary to attain this derived behavior, and because the fossil record of hominid evolution shows the evolution of these skeletal features (Wood, 1992). The supposition that early hominids had the neural capacity necessary for walking is reasonable, since chimpanzees can walk upright for short periods (Goodall, 1986). This observation leads to the reasonable inference that early hominids also had this level of neural capacity. Therefore, biological anthropologists believe that early hominids were walking upright, though not as efficiently as modern humans, at least 4 million years ago (White, Suwu, and Asfaw, 1994).

We face at least two problems in applying similar techniques to study the evolution of language or complex aspects of human behavior such as morality. First, the soft tissue of the brain is not preserved in the fossil record; and second, it would be difficult to deduce the linguistic or cognitive capacities of an extinct hominid even if we had a fossil brain, because gross anatomy does not signify function. As was noted in Chapter 4, vocal output is unaffected by stimulation or ablation of areas of the monkey neocortex, whereas similar procedures in these areas disrupt human speech (Ojemann and Mateer, 1979; MacLean and Newman, 1988; Sutton and Jergens, 1988; Ojemann et al., 1989). Although some studies have stated that certain gross anatomical features of the human brain can be discerned that confer linguistic ability (Geschwind and Levitsky, 1968; Galaburda et al., 1985; Deacon, 1988, 1997; Williams and Wakefield, 1994), recent studies, reviewed below, show that these claims do not hold.

Evolutionary Psychology

One approach to this seemingly intractable problem is that advocated by the practitioners of "evolutionary psychology" (Tooby and Cosmides, 1992). Evolutionary psychology, which derives from Wilson's (1975) "sociobiological" theory, proposes that human behavior is determined by innate, genetically transmitted neural mechanisms. The proposition is reasonable insofar as our genes do influence some aspects of human behavior. Kagan et al. (1988), for example, show that shyness depends in part on genetically transmitted traits. Kagan reached this conclusion by studying hundreds of children and their parents over more than forty years (Kagan, 1989). However, evolutionary psychologists wish to account for many other aspects of human social behavior, such as family organization, courtship, and morality, for which no equivalent data base exists. The shortcut they adopt is to imagine how our distant ancestors lived. Scenarios are proposed that are superficially "Darwinian," insofar as they claim that natural selection occurred, yielding particular genetically determined behaviors that enhanced biological fitness.

A typical example is the scenario proposed by Derek Bickerton for the evolution of syntax. Bickerton's story focuses on how males supposedly obtained mates in the Pleistocene (Bickerton, 1998b; Calvin and Bickerton, 2000). Bickerton replaces the familiar cartoon caveman dragging a female by her hair with a longer story. According to Bickerton, our ancestors lived in bands in which all females were the sexual property of an "alpha male." Other males desiring females banded together. While some lesser males distracted the alpha male, another one would couple with a willing female. Reciprocal altruism monitored by a hypothetical "cheater-detector" gene was then, according to Bickerton, the preadaptive basis for the basic aspects of syntax and the hypothetical genetically transmitted "Universal Grammar" proposed by Chomsky. No comparative evidence supports this scenario. We could just as well suppose that humans lived in large bands in which they mated freely so that paternity was generally unknown, as is the case in present-day chimpanzees (Goodall, 1986), or that the nuclear family has a long evolutionary past, based on genes that enhance biological fitness, a plausible story since fathers usually bond with their children and protect them. We also could provide a different conclusion to Bickerton's scenario, in which a lesser male kills the alpha male, ascending to supremacy. That ending would better match recorded human behavior, the historical record of assassinations, patricide, and military coups. Or we could propose a Casanova scenario in which silver-tongued seducers increased their biological fitness, thereby selecting for genes that enhance linguistic ability. In truth we can argue for a genetic basis for virtually any aspect of human behavior—greed, envy, lust, altruism, or morality—by inventing a suitable story about life in the Pleistocene.[1]

Moreover, one of Darwin's insights was his adoption of the principle of "uniformitarianism," borrowed from the geological studies of his time (Mayr, 1982). Darwin adopted the principle that, absent evidence to the contrary, one should assume that the conditions of life in the past were similar to those in the present. It is obvious that human societies differ profoundly in our own time. The effects of culture and tradition transcend genetic endowment—the children of Asian and European immigrants to the Americas act in manners far more similar to each other than to their ancestral cultures. There is no reason to suppose that genetic determinism governed human behavior in past epochs. In short, no evidence appears to support the presence of a "cheater-detector" gene or a "morality" gene (Wright, 1994). The rapid changes in moral conduct that mark human societies (the transformation in one generation of the Mongols from ruthless butchers into devout Buddhists, of Vikings into Scandinavians, the mass murder of the Nazi era) would not be possible if human morality really were genetically determined (Lieberman, 1998).

Chomskian "Evolutionary" Models of Language

The dominant linguistic theories of the day owe much to Noam Chomsky's work. It is therefore not surprising to find questions posed and solutions proposed for the evolution of key elements of his theories. For reasons that are not entirely clear, Chomsky for many years (1976, 1980a, 1980b, 1986) claimed that human linguistic ability could not have evolved by means of Darwinian processes. Chomsky's position perhaps derives from his belief that language is a faculty that is completely independent of other aspects of human behavior. In earlier versions of his theory, Chomsky proposed that humans possessed an innate, species-specific "language-acquisition device" that enabled children to acquire the rules of grammar. Later formulations of his theories proposed an innate Universal Grammar that contained specific information concerning the possible syntax of all human languages (Chomsky, 1986). The balance between the syntactic information coded in the lexicon and by algorithmic "rules" varies in various formulations of Chomsky's theories, but the necessary information is presumed to be genetically transmitted.

Bickerton, who accepts the proposition that human linguistic ability, especially syntactic ability, derives from an innate "organ" instantiating a Universal Grammar, connected these two elements in his 1990 theory for the evolution of language. He proposed a sudden mutation that restructured the human brain, creating syntactic ability all of a piece by means of neural connections between the sites in the brain in which he believed that words were represented. However, he presented no neurobiological data that supported this speculation. Models that posit unspecified sudden mutations yielding syntax have been proposed by Newmeyer (1991) and Burling (1993). Piatelli-Palmarini (1989) linked the appearance of human language to a cognitive base and some sudden unspecified mutations or mutation (or a fortuitous secondary "exaptation") that yielded one or more of the attributes—an extensive vocabulary, speech, syntax—that differentiated human language from the communications of other living primates.

Pinker and Bloom (1990) and Pinker (1994) instead argue that Universal Grammar evolved by means of natural selection from some unspecified neural structures. However, since they do not identify the neural structures that were modified to yield the Universal Grammar, specifically rejecting neural mechanisms regulating motor control, it is difficult to evaluate their theory. Pinker (1994, p. 353), moreover, adopts a neophrenological position, equating Broca's area with human linguistic ability. Bloom (personal communication) suggests that the preadaptive base for the evolution of the UG might have been some unspecified part of the hominid brain that served no function whatsoever. Hence, the hypothetical UG could be morphologically and functionally independent of the neuroanatomical structures regulating other aspects of behavior. The burden of proof is on Bloom to provide evidence supporting the claim that *any* structure exists in the brain of any animal that has no function whatsoever. Williams and Wakefield (1994) claim that UG was present in the brains of *Homo erectus,* perhaps in earlier *Homo habilis* hominids. Their claim (discussed below) is based on inferences from endocasts of fossil skulls, which supposedly reveal the presence of Broca's and Wernicke's areas and adjacent cortical regions that in turn supposedly reveal linguistic ability. They also claim that stone tool technology supposedly reveals fully formed language 1.5 million years ago.

Calvin and Bickerton (2000) propose that sexual activity, cheater-detector genes, and reciprocal altruism were some of the preadaptive bases for language. Calvin again proposes that neural connections between words stored in sites in the temporal lobe instantiate the Universal Grammar. However, Calvin's argument for motor control's being the preadaptive basis for the evolutionary process that ultimately yielded the neural substrate of Universal Grammar is not consistent with neurophysiologic data or the principles of evolutionary biology. It owes more to Lamarck than to Darwin, invoking "soft" inheritance, the transmission of phenotypically acquired characteristics to one's progeny. Calvin (1993) claims that human beings uniquely possess the cortical brain mechanisms that allow us to throw projectiles forcefully and accurately. Calvin argues that these cortical mechanisms constitute the bases for the evolution of human linguistic and cognitive ability. His evolutionary claims hinge on a scenario in which early hominids hunted by throwing sharpened stones. But it is obvious that very few people can hit a target when they forcefully hurl a ball, let alone a stone. Accurate missile throwing is an acquired skill. As noted in Chapter 1, neurophysiologic studies (e.g., Evarts, 1973; Sanes and Donoghue, 1996, 1997, in press) show that neural circuits regulating motor control are shaped as an animal or human learns to execute specific motor acts. In other words, there is no genetically predetermined store of motor commands that constitutes a "Universal Motor Control Grammar." Therefore, the biological mechanism proposed by Calvin and Bickerton for a Universal Grammar would entail Lamarckian soft inheritance, a process that is outside the domain of modern biological thought (Mayr, 1982).

Universal Grammar

Nor, despite Steven Pinker's (1994) claim, is there any evidence for a gene for Universal Grammar. Pinker cited Gopnick and Crago's (1991) account of the supposed linguistic deficits caused by a genetic anomaly in three generations of a large extended family (Family KE). Gopnick and Crago claimed that afflicted family members were unable to produce the regular past tense of English verbs and regular plurals of English nouns, though their command of irregular verbs and nouns was supposedly unimpaired. Gopnick and Crago also claimed that the afflicted members of the family had no cognitive deficits. This is not the case (Vargha-Khudem et al., 1995, 1998). The behavioral deficits of the afflicted members of this family do have a genetic basis (Fisher et al., 1998). However, Vargha-Khadem et al. (1998) show that the primary deficit of these individuals is

> an impairment in sequential articulation (i.e., a verbal dyspraxia) so severe that the speech of the affected members is often rendered incomprehensible to the naive listener. This articulatory disorder [yields] an impairment in nonspeech movements as well. The disorder is not restricted to orofacial movements and articulation but also extends to both expressive and to a lesser degree to receptive language abilities. Furthermore, the afflicted family members show significant deficits not only in verbal intelligence but also in nonverbal intelligence such that the full-scale intelligence quotients of the affected individuals (7 of the 13 tested) fall below the low average range (80–89), with two only scoring 81. In contrast, none of the unaffected family members had full-scale intelligence quotients below the low average range. (P. 12695)

MRIs of the affected family members' brains revealed cortical damage in some of the afflicted individuals. However, the major finding was bilateral reduction in the volume of a basal ganglia structure: both left- and right-hemisphere caudate nucleus were significantly smaller in the afflicted group than in the unafflicted group. It is therefore not surprising that the sequencing deficits of Family KE resemble those noted by Pickett et al. (1998) for a subject having bilateral damage to the putamen and the head of the caudate nucleus.

Vargha-Khadem and her colleagues conclude:

> The same developing neural network controlling oromotor coordination and expressive language may also be a prerequisite for the emergence of "inner speech" and the development of higher-order thought processes, in which case a central abnormality affecting speech production could have a cascading effect resulting in intellectual deficits. According to this view, the multiple behavioral impairments of the affected family members might all be traceable to abnormality of a single neural network basic to speech production. (1998, p. 12700)

In short, the deficits of Family KE demonstrate that the neural capacity for human language has an innate, genetic basis. However, their behavioral deficits in all likelihood derive from impairment of the striatal components of the functional language system.

A Darwinian Model for the Evolution of Language

In the model that follows I propose that human language has different biological components, some primitive, some derived. Lexical ability and the ability to comprehend simple aspects of syntax can be observed in living apes, which in all likelihood retain some of the neural attributes of the extinct 5-million-year-old common ancestor of humans and apes. Ape-human lexical and syntactic abilities differ, but are quantitative. Apes can produce about 150 words using manual sign language or computer keyboards, roughly equivalent to the abilities of two year-old children. Humans typically have vocabularies exceeding 10,000 words. Although syntactic ability is usually taken to be the hallmark of "true" human language (e.g., Bickerton, 1990, 1998b; Calvin and Bickerton, 2000), chimpanzees also can comprehend simple signed or spoken sentences, again roughly equivalent to the abilities of two year-old children. The limits of lexical and syntactic ability in apes and human children are roughly equal, since grammar does not really take off in children until vocabulary exceeds 250 words (Bates and Goodman, 1997). In contrast, fluent speech, the ability to produce novel sound sequences that signal words, appears to be the product of species-specific attributes of the human brain. Apes never learn to talk. This human capacity may reflect subcortical basal ganglia function.

Chimpanzee Language

Although chimpanzees are not hominids, they are the closest living approximations to the common human-chimpanzee ancestor (McGrew, 1993), and arguably are the best starting point for the study of the evolution of the neural bases of human language. We can narrow the search for the properties that set human language apart from whatever capacities exist in chimpanzees and other animals. Moreover, the data from these studies refute theories that claim that human language is the result of a singular mutation that yielded full-blown human language (Bickerton, 1990) or the secondary result of evolution for some other unspecified aspect of behavior (Piatelli-Palmarini, 1989; Pinker and Bloom, 1990; Bloom, personal communication).

Normal human children reared in any normal situation usually start to talk before the third year of life. Conversely, children raised without exposure to language never develop normal linguistic or normal cognitive ability. And those individuals suffering from extreme forms of mental retardation never develop language (Wills, 1973). For example, the degree of retardation in Down's syndrome varies from slight incapacity to profound mental retardation requiring institutional care; these individuals never acquire normal language in any situation (Benda, 1969). Therefore, exposure to a normal human childrearing environment is a necessary and sufficient condition for the acquisition of language, *if* the neural substrate necessary for language is present. This being the case, it is possible to assess the linguistic potential of the chimpanzee brain by rearing chimpanzees in a human environment.

The first cross-fostering chimpanzee language experiment that met with success was directed by Beatrix and Alan Gardner. The Gardners proposed to see what would happen if a chimpanzee was raised as though it were human in a linguistic environment using American Sign Language (ASL). The Gardners' (1969) project commenced with the ten-month-old female chimpanzee Washoe who lived with the Gardners and their research team from

1966 to 1970. During that period she was treated as though she was a child, albeit one who was in contact with an adult during all of her waking hours. She was clothed, wore shoes, learned to use cups, spoons, and the toilet, and played with toys. She observed ASL conversations between adults and communications in ASL directed toward her, without the adults' necessarily expecting her to understand what was being signed in the early stages of the project. Washoe acquired about 50 ASL words in the first year of cross-fostering. In November 1972 four newborn chimpanzees, Moja, Pili, Tatu, and Dar, were placed in four adoptive "families" at the Gardners' laboratory. One or more of the human members of each family remained with each chimpanzee from 7:00 A.M. to 8:00 P.M. throughout the year. Each family had one or more people who were proficient in ASL. Records of the chimpanzees' ASL productions were kept; the chimpanzees' ASL vocabularies were also formally tested (Gardner and Gardner, 1984). In the first two years the chimpanzees' ASL vocabularies reached 50 signs, a performance roughly equivalent to that of either hearing human children or deaf children raised from birth onward in homes using ASL.

However, the performance of the chimpanzees and human children diverges after age two. When the Gardners' project ended the chimpanzees had a vocabulary of about 140 words after 60 months of cross-fostered life. The rate at which they had acquired words, about 3 signs per month, was about the same over the entire period. In marked contrast, once normal children raised under normal conditions approach age three, it generally becomes very difficult to keep track of the number of words they know. A "naming explosion" occurs concurrently with increased grammatical ability.

These findings have been replicated by Savage-Rumbaugh and Rumbaugh using somewhat different cross-fostering techniques and a visual-manual communication system at the Yerkes Language Research Center. The linguistic behavior of Kanzi, a Bonobo or pygmy chimpanzee, has been noted in many publications and films. The published evidence (Savage-Rumbaugh and Rumbaugh, 1993) indicates that Kanzi's abilities, though superior to those of the other "common" chimpanzees (*Pan troglodytes*) at Yerkes, are on a par with those of Tatu, the most proficient of the Project Washoe chimpanzees. Kanzi, like the Project Washoe chimpanzees, uses toys, goes on excursions with his human family members, and is engaged in conversations directed to him. In contrast to Project Washoe, Kanzi's human companions talk to each other and to him in English. Kanzi's "utterances" are formed as he points to "lexigrams" on boards or computer terminals. Each lexigram represents an English word and can, when Kanzi is using a terminal connected to a speech synthesizer, trigger the English word that corresponds to the lexigram. Using somewhat different methods, the Yerkes research group replicated the Project Washoe (Gardner and Gardner, 1984) findings on the referential nature of Kanzi's vocabulary. The lexigrams represent concepts that correspond to the words that form the vocabularies of young human children. Kanzi at age six seems to have about the same linguistic ability as the five-year-old Project Washoe chimpanzees.

The lexical capacities of human beings and chimpanzees clearly differ. However, chimpanzees can invent new words and can combine words to form new words (Gardner and Gardner, 1984; Savage-Rumbaugh et al., 1986; Savage-Rumbaugh and Rumbaugh, 1993). For example, they spontaneously form new words by compounding old words, forming *waterbird*—duck, from the semantically distinct words *water* and *bird* (Gardner, Gardner, and Van Cantfort, 1989).[2] Chimpanzees also can understand spoken English words (Gardner and Gardner, 1984, in press; Gardner, Gardner, and Van Cantfort, 1989; Savage-Rumbaugh and Rumbaugh, 1993). Indeed, other animals comprehend spoken words. Domesticated dogs almost always comprehend a few words. The celebrated circus dog Fellow comprehended at least 50 words (Warden and Warner, 1928). Lexical ability dissociated from speech production is therefore a primitive feature of human language that undoubtedly existed in archaic hominids.

Syntax and "Protolanguage"

Syntactic ability, which was and still is taken to be a unique human attribute (Lieberman, 1975, 1984, 1991; Bickerton 1990, 1998b; Calvin and Bickerton, 2000) is also present to a limited degree in chimpanzees. Recent analyses of the American Sign Language (ASL) communications of the Project Washoe chimpanzees show that they productively used two sign combinations as well as some three sign combinations (Gardner and Gardner, 1994). The Gardners' cross-fostered chimpanzees also productively used the inflected forms of their ASL signs, though in a manner similar to that of young deaf children. The ASL sign for *quiet* is, for example, formed on the signer's lips; movement toward some person indicates the object of the verb. The cross-fostered chimpanzees would instead place the hand gesture that forms the sign on the lips of the person or chimpanzee who was supposed to be quiet. The cross-fostered Gardner chimpanzees, in other words, command some aspects of morphophonemics. The cross-fostered bonobo Kanzi, whose linguistic input is spoken English, performed slightly better than a two-year-old child in a test in which he had to carry out various activities that were requested by spoken sentences. Neither the two-year-old child nor Kanzi demonstrated comprehension of moderately complex English syntax. However, the six-year-old chimpanzee's responses indicated that he had mastered the canonical form of English in which the subject (or omitted subject) always precedes the object. Kanzi responded correctly about 75 percent of the time when he heard sentences such as *Put the pine needles on the ball* and *Put the ball on the pine needles.* Kanzi placed either the pine needles on the ball or the ball on the pine needles in response to the appropriate English-language command, demonstrating a sensitivity to basic word order in English.

In comprehending the meaning of these sentences, Kanzi also met a litmus test proposed by Derek Bickerton that supposedly reveals the presence of true "language" rather than "protolanguage." According to Bickerton (1990, 1998b), protolanguage consists of strings of words that lack syntactic structure. In contrast, "true" language employs syntax; Bickerton concludes that the mark of a mind that can command syntax is the fact that adults and older children can "recover" the omitted subject "you" in sentences such as *Put the pine needles on the ball.* Apparently, Bickerton believes that the syntactic relations between the words of the sentence are the sole factors guiding the listener or reader toward the recovery of the omitted word. Bickerton ignores the role of pragmatic context. However, since Kanzi comprehends the command *Put the pine needles on the ball,* we must conclude that Bickerton's test shows that the bonobo possess the neural substrate that governs "true" language. Bickerton predictably rejects this evidence of chimpanzee syntactic ability. His "solution" to the dilemma that chimpanzees might possess true language is a peculiar syntactic analysis of the sentence *Put the pine needles on the ball.* Bickerton asserts that "these commands don't contain any subjects, they show objects preceding prepositional phrases of place" (1998a). Bickerton simply avoids addressing the fact that Kanzi made use of syntactic word order to carry out the requested action.

A distinction between "protolanguage" and "true" language based on syntax appears to be unproductive, since there does not appear to be a sharp dichotomy between having syntax or not. The limited syntactic abilities of chimpanzees may be related to their ability to produce and comprehend a limited number of words. The relationship between syntax and lexical ability may not be fortuitous. The data of Bates and Goodman (1997) show that the development of syntactic and lexical abilities in children cannot be dissociated; a strong correlation exists between vocabulary size and the acquisition of syntax in young children. English-speaking children who can produce 150 words also begin to produce syntactically connected utterances. This finding is not surprising, since a child's passive receptive vocabulary is generally about six times greater than its productive vocabulary. Therefore, children who are able to speak only 150 words can comprehend about 900 words, including the grammatical "function" words of English. Indeed, as Bates and Goodman point out, a distinction between protolanguage and language based on syntax no longer seems justified on theoretical grounds. The distinction between syntax and the lexicon is blurred in Chomsky's (1995) "minimalist" theory and has essentially disappeared in "construction grammar" (Fillmore et al., 1988; Goldberg, 1995). In these linguistic theories, the lexicon captures grammatical distinctions formerly considered to be processed in an independent "syntactic" component. Moreover, the distinction between syntax and the lexicon formerly posited by theoretical linguists focusing on English obviously does not exist in highly inflected languages such as Sanskrit, classical Greek, and American Sign Language or in contemporary languages such as Italian (Stokie, 1978; Bates and Goodman, 1997).

Since chimpanzees possess limited syntactic ability, it would be surprising if early hominids such as the Australopithecines lacked any syntactic ability. Therefore, it is most improbable that syntactic ability suddenly developed, as Bickerton (1990) proposed, in the ice ages, when our ancestors supposedly conquered the Neanderthals,[3] or in the Upper Paleololithic (Davidson and Noble, 1993). Nor is it likely that advanced syntactic ability was possessed only by anatomically modern *Homo sapiens* 150,000 years or so in the past (Lieberman, 1991). A gradual development of syntactic ability over the course of hominid evolution seems most likely for the reasons that will be discussed below. The gradual development of language proposed by Aiello and Dunbar (1993) is plausible, but not by the mechanism that they propose. Aiello and Dunbar link neocortical volume to group size and language to neocortical size. However, although the data that they present to support an expansion of the neocortex keyed to the size of a primate social community generally fit their theory, one crucial data point is missing that refutes their theory—the large neocortex of solitary Orangutans.

Human Language and Speech

Chimpanzees cannot talk. Hayes and Hayes (1951) raised the infant chimpanzee Viki as though it were a human child. The chimpanzee was exposed both to normal human conversation and to the "motherese" variety of speech commonly directed toward young children (Fernald et al., 1989). Despite intensive speech training, Viki could produce only four human words that were barely intelligible when the project ended because of Viki's death at age seven years. Viki's inability to speak is consistent with Goodall's observations of chimpanzees in their natural habitat. Goodall notes: "Chimpanzee vocalizations are closely bound to emotion. The production of a sound in the *absence* of the appropriate emotional state seems to be an almost impossible task for a chimpanzee . . . Chimpanzees can learn to *suppress* calls in situations when the production of sounds might, by drawing attention to the signaler, place him in an unpleasant or dangerous situation, but even this is not easy" (1986, p. 125). It is clear that chimpanzees cannot even produce vocalizations that are not "bound" to specific emotional states (Lieberman, 1994a). Therefore, speech is a derived feature of human language.

The Antiquity of Speech

However, this does not mean that speech is a recent feature of hominid evolution. Purposeful, referential speech must have existed well before the evolution of anatomically modern *Homo sapiens.* The basis for this conclusion paradoxically rests in the claim that the anatomy necessary to produce the full range of human speech was absent in *Homo erectus* and certain, if not all, Neanderthals.

The anatomical basis for the modulation of formant frequencies that is one of the central characteristics of human speech is the airway above the larynx. The human upper airway that constitutes the supralaryngeal vocal tract (SVT) differs from that of all other living species (Negus, 1949; Lieberman, 1968). Although the human SVT enhances the process of speech perception, it also *decreases* biological fitness by making swallowing liquids and solid food more risky. The only biological function that the human SVT appears to enhance is the saliency of speech sounds (Lieberman, 1975, 1984, 1991, 1998; Laitman, Heimbuch, and Crelin, 1979; Carré et al., 1994; Hauser, 1996; D. Lieberman, 1998).

Figure 5-1 shows the head and neck of a young adult male chimpanzee. The tongue is positioned within the mouth. The larynx is positioned close to the base of the skull and, like the periscope of a submarine, can be raised to form a passageway in which air flows through the nose into the chimpanzee's lungs, sealed off from the flow of liquids and small particles of food that can simultaneously pass to either side of the raised larynx into the pharynx and from there to the digestive tract. All nonhuman primates and newborn human beings possess the standard-plan supralaryngeal airway (Negus, 1949). Victor Negus (1949) also pointed out the advantages of this standard-plan airway for breathing and swallowing. Since the larynx can remain in this raised position except when large pieces of food are swallowed, an animal can breathe and drink or ingest small pieces of food without the possi-

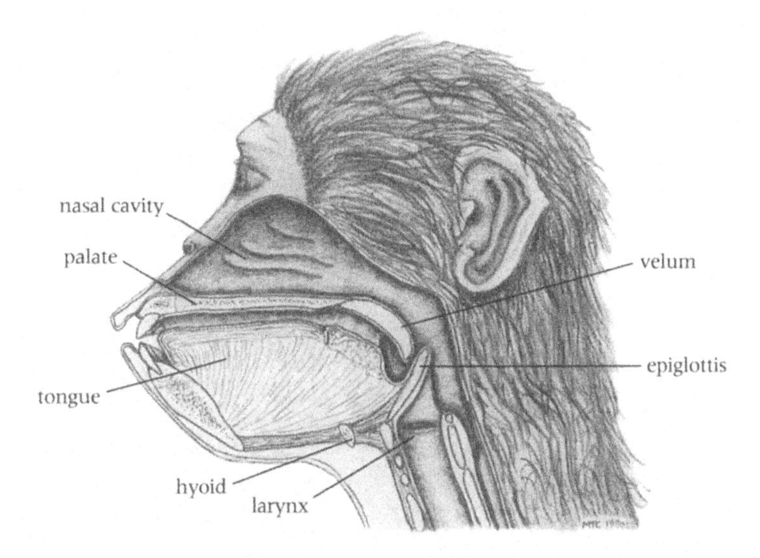

Figure 5-1. The head and neck of an adult male chimpanzee. Note the high position of the larynx, the long oral cavity, and the position of the tongue in the mouth.

bility of food or drink entering the larynx or lungs. Liquids and small pieces of solid food pass to either side of the larynx while it is locked into the nose. Liquids and food particles are then propelled down the pharynx, which is positioned behind the animal's larynx.

Figure 5-2 shows the human supralaryngeal configuration. The larynx occupies a low position relative to the mandible and vertebrae of the spinal column; it cannot lock into the nasal cavity. Normal swallowing in humans is achieved through a sequence of coordinated maneuvers of the tongue, the jaw, the pharyngeal constrictor muscles, and muscles that move the hyoid bone. In humans the superior pharyngeal constrictor muscle propels substances down the pharynx (Palmer and Hiiemae, 1997; Palmer, Hiiemae, and Liu, 1997). The larynx must be pulled forward so that food and drink enter the digestive tract. If not, a person can choke to death if food lodges in the larynx. The odd morphology and negative consequences of the adult human supralaryngeal vocal tract (SVT) were known to Charles Darwin, who noted the "strange fact that every particle of food and drink which we

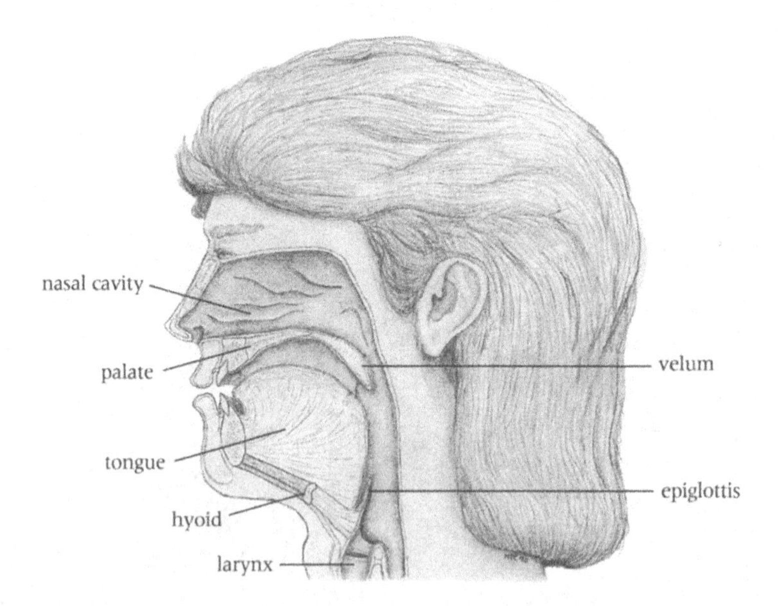

Figure 5-2. Lateral view of an adult human supralaryngeal vocal tract (SVT). Note the low position of the larynx, the comparatively short human mouth, and the shape of the human tongue. The human SVT has an oral cavity and pharynx of almost equal length.

swallow has to pass over the orifice of the trachea, with some risk of falling into the lungs" (1859, p. 191).

Note the posterior, almost circular contour of the tongue in Figure 5-2. The horizontal oral cavity and vertically oriented pharynx are almost equal in length. The shape of the tongue is scarcely altered when the different vowels of English are produced (Russell, 1928; Carmody, 1937; Chiba and Kajiyama, 1941; Perkell, 1969; Ladefoged et al., 1972; Nearey, 1979; Baer et al., 1991; Story et al., 1996). Radiographic studies of vowel production in other languages show similar results (Chiba and Kajiyama, 1941; Fant, 1960; Ladefoged et al., 1972). The contour of the tongue forms two "tubes," a horizontal "tube" formed by the human mouth and a vertical pharynx "tube." Abrupt changes in the cross-sectional areas of these tubes can be formed by simply moving the tongue body forward or backward and up or down. The approximately equal lengths of the two tubes make it possible to produce the "quantal" or "point" vowels [i], [u], and [a] (Stevens, 1972; Beckman et al., 1995). These vowels have spectral peaks because two formant frequencies converge (Stevens and House, 1955; Fant, 1960; Stevens, 1972, Carré et al., 1994). These spectral-peak vowels, auditory analogues of saturated colors, are acoustically salient (Lindblom, 1966, 1988). They are the most common vowels among human languages (Jakobson, 1940; Greenberg, 1963). Children make fewer errors when they learn words that contain these vowels (Olmsted, 1971). The error rates for [i] and [u] are lowest for adults (Peterson and Barney, 1952) owing to the fact that these vowels, particularly [i], provide an optimal signal for vocal tract normalization (Nearey, 1979; Fitch, 1994, 1997).

A 1971 study by Lieberman and Crelin that attempted to reconstruct the SVT of the La Chapelle-aux-Saints Neanderthal fossil noted that the fossil's skull base, the basicranium, resembled that of a large newborn human infant; the reconstructed Neanderthal SVT, like a human newborn's, was incapable of producing the vowels [i], [u], or [a] (Lieberman et al., 1972). The two factors that precluded its being able to produce these sounds were that the oral cavity of the La Chapelle-aux-Saints Neanderthal was much longer than that of any modern human adult (Howells, 1979, 1989), and the La Chapelle-aux-Saints larynx was judged to be positioned close to the base of its skull similar to that of a human newborn. These two factors yielded an SVT in which the oral cavity was very long and the pharynx short, making it impossible to produce quantal vowels. Computer-modeling studies show that it is impossible to produce these vowels absent an SVT with an oral cavity and pharynx roughly equal in length (Lieberman, 1968; Lieberman et al., 1969; Lieberman and Crelin, 1971; Lieberman, Crelin, and Klatt, 1972; Carré et al., 1994).

Crelin's 1971 reconstruction followed the principles of comparative anatomy, inferring similar relationships between skeletal morphology and soft tissue in closely related species. The principles and data of recent studies support Crelin's inferences. Alberch (1989) has advanced the principles of "dev-ev," a process wherein divergences in the path of evolution of related species can be understood by studying their ontogenetic development. As Darwin (1859) noted, related species that have different characteristics as adults often resemble each other to a greater degree in their infantile stages. The derived features that differentiate these species appear as they mature. Studies such as Vleck (1970) show that the skulls of young Neanderthal fossils bear a closer resemblance to present-day humans than the skulls of older Neanderthal children and adolescents. The Neanderthal face appears to follow the growth pattern of living apes; their faces project forward, anterior to their foreheads. The Neanderthal growth pattern, like those of apes, yields a long mouth. In contrast, recent studies show that the human face's growth pattern diverges from the general primate pattern. Through a process of differential bone growth, the human face instead moves backward (D. Lieberman, 1998). By the end of the first year of life the human skull base is flexed compared to those of Neanderthals and apes (Laitman, Heimbuch, and Crelin, 1979; Laitman and Heimbuch, 1982). During the next five years of life the human larynx descends relative to the vertebral column and mandible (D. Lieberman and McCarthy, 1999). The restructuring of the human skull base, in which the face moves back so that it is in line with the upper cranium, yields the relatively short human mouth. The descent of the larynx yields the long human pharynx. The net result is the human SVT, in which the oral cavity and pharynx have almost the same length. Since the first phase of this process does not occur in Neanderthals (Vleck, 1970; D. Lieberman, 1998), it is reasonable to assume that the second phase, the descent of the larynx, also does not occur. Moreover, an additional fact argues against classic Neanderthals' having a human SVT; the long Neanderthal mouth would have to be matched by an equally long pharynx, placing the larynx in the Neanderthal chest (Lieberman, 1984, 1991), unlike any living hominoid.

However, as Lieberman and Crelin (1971) stressed, their study did not demonstrate that Neanderthals lacked speech. In fact they explicitly stated that Neanderthals must have possessed language and speech. Neanderthal speech simply was not as efficient a medium of vocal communication as human speech. This conclusion follows from the logic of natural selection: the restructuring of the human SVT to enhance the perception of speech would not have contributed to biological fitness *unless* speech and language were already present in the hominid species ancestral to modern *Homo sapiens*. Otherwise there would have been no reason for the retention of the lower laryngeal position of the human SVT. Therefore, speech and language must have already been present in *Homo erectus* and in Neanderthals. This was pointed out in the initial Lieberman and Crelin (1971) paper on Neanderthal speech capabilities.[4] Although many subsequent studies have cited this paper to support the position that speech and language were absent in Neanderthals (e.g., Davidson and Noble, 1993), limits on phonetic ability do not signify the absence of speech and language.

Critiques of the Lieberman and Crelin (1971) SVT reconstruction have claimed that the lower position of the human larynx and the hyoid bone (which supports the larynx) is a necessary condition for swallowing in upright hominids (Falk, 1975; Houghton, 1993; Schepartz, 1993). According to this view, upright bipedal hominids, including Neanderthals, would have had to have a low humanlike larynx position, yielding a long humanlike pharynx.[5] This argument rested on the theory that the mechanics of human swallowing differed profoundly from those of other mammals. However, recent studies show that tongue and jaw movements in humans are linked during feeding as they are in other mammals (Palmer and Hiiemae, 1997; Palmer, Hiiemae, and Liu, 1997). The radiographic studies of Jeffrey Palmer and his colleagues show that upright bipedal hominids can swallow with a high hyoid similar to that of a chimpanzee. Therefore, it is incorrect to claim that the human SVT (which has a low larynx position) evolved to make swallowing possible. The only adaptive value of the low human larynx appears to be to enhance the phonetic robustness of human speech. The larynx gradually descends from birth onward in human children reaching a position that creates an SVT that has a pharynx and oral cavity of equal length between ages five and six years. As children continue to grow, the length of the pharynx continues to match the length of the oral cavity, preserving the "quantal" speech production conditions noted above (D, Lieberman, 1998).[6] The neural mechanism that allows human listeners to determine the length of the SVT of the person whose speech they are "decoding" (Liberman et al., 1967) appears to be innate, since it is in place by age three months (Lieberman, 1984). However, the ability to infer the length of a person's SVT from speech is not a derived human trait; comparative studies of monkeys show that they judge the length of another monkey's SVT—which is a good index of its size—by a similar process (Fitch, 1994, 1997).[7] Therefore, early hominids must have possessed this ability. Moreover, nonhuman primate calls are differentiated through the formant frequency patterns generated when monkeys or apes close or open their lips as they phonate (Lieberman, 1968, 1975). The use of formant frequency patterns to communicate information is not limited to primates. The pioneering studies of Frishkopf and Goldstein (1963) and Capranica (1965) showed that the mating calls of different species of frogs are differentiated by formant frequency patterns.

The fundamental frequency of phonation (F0), which is determined by laryngeal muscles and alveolar (lung) air pressure, is one of the principal cues that signals the end of a sentence and major syntactic units (Armstrong and Ward, 1926; Lieberman, 1967). Most human languages make use of controlled variations of F0 to produce "tones" that differentiate words (Greenberg, 1963). Since apes possess laryngeal anatomy that can generate F0 contours (Negus, 1949), early hominids must have had this ability. In other words, the roots of speech communication may extend back to the earliest phases of hominid evolution.

When Did the FLS Evolve?

A review of the fossil and archaeological record reveals that a gradual increase in the size of the hominid brain occurred and that tools became more complex over time. But the question that must concern us here is what inferences we can make from this evidence concerning the evolution of the FLS.

Walking and Basal Ganglia

About 5 million years ago a species lived that was the common ancestor of present-day apes and humans (Sarich, 1974). The remains of the common ancestral species have not yet been found, but early hominid fossils have been uncovered, such as the 4.4-million-year-old *Ardipithecus ramidus.* These hominids greatly resemble apes, but they possessed anatomy that enabled them to walk upright, though less efficiently than later hominids (White,

Suwu, and Asfaw, 1994; Leakey et al., 1995). The 3.6-million-year-old *Australopithecus afarensis* fossils unearthed in Ethiopia (one was named "Lucy") had similar anatomy adapted for upright bipedal locomotion. Australopithecine-grade fossils had small brains. The volume of their brains, as estimated from the internal volume of their crania, ranges between 350 and 530 cc, somewhat larger than the average 400-cc brains of present-day chimpanzees (Wood, 1992). Bipedalism, which can be inferred from the fossils' bones (the lower limbs, the pelvis, the orientation of the spinal column and head, and the spinal column itself), had consequences beyond locomotion.

Upright bipedal locomotion may have been the preadaptive factor that selected for neural mechanisms that enhanced motor ability (Jesse Hochstadt, personal communication). It is apparent that human beings *learn* to walk. The "walking reflex" that exists in newborn human infants appears to be controlled by a *quadripedal* neural "pattern generator" that reflects our hominoid ancestry (Thelen, 1984). In contrast to colts, whose innate quadripedal motor-control programs enable them to run shortly after birth, humans go through a long process learning to locomote bipedally. Apart from the fact that human infants are "large, fat, weak and unstable" (Thelen, 1984, p. 246), they have to override this archaic quadripedal motor program for walking. The process is protracted, and we crawl and toddle before we are able to walk or run without lurching and falling. Heel strike, which marks efficient bipedal locomotion, takes years to develop. The subcortical basal ganglia structures that are crucial components of the FLS regulate upright, bipedal locomotion. Indeed one of the primary signs of Parkinson's disease, in which basal ganglia circuits are degraded, is impaired locomotion (Hoehn and Yahr, 1967). Thus, it is quite possible that upright, bipedal locomotion was the initial selective force for the enhancement of the subcortical sequencing ability that marks both motor control and cognition.

Manual Dexterity

Walking freed hominid hands to carry objects and manipulate tools. The fossil record shows that some Australopithecines who lived during this period possessed another derived hominid feature, fingers that are adapted to precise, forceful manual activity—the human "power grip" (Sussman, 1994). Primitive stone "Oldowan" tools that can be dated to approximately 2.5 million years ago have been found in African sites (Semaw et al., 1997); some undated stone tools may be older. The name Oldowan refers to one of the sites at which these tools were first found, the Olduvai Gorge, Tanzania. However, similar tools dated to the same era have been found in Kenya, Ethiopia, Algeria, and South Africa. Oldowan tools appear to be simple—they are stones from which sections have been flaked away—but they require skills that have never been observed in present-day apes. As Toth and Schick (1993) note, the hominids who made these tools had

> (a) the ability to recognize acute angles on cores [the piece of stone from which a tool is flaked off] to serve as striking platforms from which to detach flakes and fragments, and (b) good hand-eye coordination when flaking stone, including the dexterity to strike the core with a hammerstone with a sharp, glancing blow. It would appear that a strong power grip, as well as a strong precision grip, was characteristic of early hominid toolmaking. (P. 349)

Oldowan tools provide some other clues to their maker's cognitive ability. Toth and Schick (1993) note that raw stock for the tools was transported over long distances. Chimpanzees have not been observed transporting material for toolmaking, so this may imply planning (a dorsolateral-prefrontal-striatal circuit function) that transcends that of chimpanzees. Oldowan tools also appear to have been made by right-handed individuals, implying left-hemisphere dominance for language.

Brain Lateralization

However, as noted in earlier chapters, brain lateralization in itself cannot be the "key" to human language. Although left-hemisphere neural structures appear to be predisposed to regulate language in about 90 percent of the present human population, right-hemisphere structures are also involved and can assume the role of left-hemisphere structures after brain damage. Moreover, it is clear that brain lateralization is a "primitive," phylogenetically ancient trait that does not indicate that an animal possesses language. It has been evident since the 1970s that the more complex aspects of birdsong are regulated by the dominant (usually the left) hemisphere of bird brains (Nottebohm and Nottebohm, 1976), but birds don't have language. As noted earlier, Bauer (1993) found that the vocalizations of frogs are regulated by one hemisphere of their brains. Frogs represent species ancestral to both birds and mammals; Bauer's frog study explains why both birds and mammals (Bradshaw and Nettleton, 1991) have lateralized brains.

For example, individual mice show paw preferences although mice as a group are not predominantly right-pawed or left-pawed. Denenberg's (1981) review of brain lateralization in animals noted examples in which one hemisphere or the other of the brain regulated the direction in which animals ran on running wheels or in left-right movements. It is also clear that human language cannot depend on having a *left*-dominant hemisphere; that would exclude millions of people who have language-dominant right hemispheres. Perhaps humans beings are usually left-hemisphere language dominant because of an evolutionary "choke point" that occurred about 5 million years ago—we are the descendants of hominids who happened to be predominantly right-handed.

Brain Expansion and Paleoneurology

Hominid fossils having brain capacities between 500 and 800 cc, almost twice the size of chimpanzees, appear in the fossil record approximately 2 million years ago. Different species classifications have been proposed for these fossils, *Homo habilis* and *Homo rudolfensis* (Wood and Collard, 1999).[8] Many archaeologists believe that these species produced the first stone tools. By 1.5 million years before the present, fossils generally classified as members of the species *Homo erectus* or *Homo ergaster* appear (Wood, 1992; Wood and Collard, 1999). Their anatomy was better adapted for bipedal locomotion; they had brain volumes ranging from 750 to 1250 cc. The "Acheulian" tools that they produced were complex, shaped and pointed symmetrical objects that have been found throughout Africa and Europe. *Homo erectus*–grade hominids established themselves throughout Europe and Asia. Other tools such as 400,000-year-old spears with fire-hardened points have been found in Europe (Thieme, 1997).

Attempts have been made to assess the language abilities of fossil hominids by determining whether their brains possessed the hypothetical "seats" of language, namely Broca's and Wernicke's areas. Apart from the debatable validity of the Lichtheim-Geschwind brain model, the claim reduces to that of determining the structure of the cortical surface of a living brain from the faint marks on endocasts (casts of the inside surface of the skulls) of fossils. The enterprise is highly speculative. The boundaries for these areas are not readily apparent when the brains of living humans are examined, which is why neurosurgeons must employ mapping techniques prior to surgery (Ojemann and Mateer, 1979; Ojemann et al., 1989). A typical speculation is the claim made by Williams and Wakefield (1994) that fully developed human language, genetically coded in a Chomksian Universal Grammar, existed in *Homo erectus,* perhaps in earlier *Homo habilis* hominids. Williams and Wakefield propose that endocasts of fossil crania reveal the presence of Broca's and Wernicke's areas and adjacent parietal-occipital-temporal cortical areas, which Williams and Wakefield equate with the brain bases of the hypothetical Chomskian Universal Grammar. However, it is improbable that these endocasts reveal the neocortical surfaces of fossil brains. As Ralph Holloway, a specialist in this field, notes, there is not one single well-documented instance of "paleoneurological evidence that unambiguously demonstrates a relative expansion of the parietal-ocipital-temporal junction in early *Homo*" (1995, p. 191).

The Evolution of Modern Human Beings

Anatomically modern human beings appear to have an African origin deriving from *Homo ergaster* (a specifically African variant of *Homo erectus*) or a related species (Wood and Collard, 1999). Both the fossil record and genetic dating techniques yield a date of between 200,000 and 100,000 years ago for the origin of modern human beings (Stringer and Andrews, 1988; Stringer, 1992; Tishkoff et al., 1996). Neanderthals are considered by many anthropologists to be a species that also evolved from *Homo erectus.* The DNA recovered from a Neanderthal fossil indicates that Neanderthals diverged from the ancestral species common to them and modern human beings somewhere between 550,000 and 690,000 years ago (Krings et al., 1997). Neanderthal fossils have been recovered that date between 200,000 and 30,000 years ago. They were first found in Europe but have since been recovered in North Africa, Israel, Iraq, and other parts of the Mideast as well as at Asian sites as far east as Uzbekistan. The opposing "multiregional" theory for human evolution claims that anatomically modern humans evolved independently in different regions of the world from indigenous *Homo erectus* populations (Frayer et al., 1993). However, reanalysis of the fossil data cited by Frayer and his colleagues to support their theory shows that it instead favors the "out-of-Africa" or "Eve" hypothesis (D. Lieberman, 1995). The brain volumes of Neanderthals and anatomically modern humans do not differ significantly, ranging up to 1500 cc. Body weight, which affects absolute brain size (Jerison, 1973; Stephan, Frahm, and Baron, 1981), is approximately equal in Neanderthals and humans.

The "Mousterian" tool technology associated with Neanderthal and contemporary anatomically modern human hominids is similar and is regarded by some specialists as an extension of lower Paleolithic techniques. Many attempts have been made to infer linguistic and cognitive ability from the archaeological record of tools and toolmaking technology. I at one time (Lieberman, 1975) suggested that the Levallois, core and flake, toolmaking technique indicated the neural capacity to acquire Chomsky's 1957 "Transformational Grammar." The "core and flake" technique is a two-stage operation. A core, which does not resemble the final product, is produced by chipping away at a rock. The desired tools are then flaked from the core by a different technique, sudden percussive blows or forceful pressure applied by a stick. I suggested that the "core" was analogous to the "deep" level postulated by Chomsky's 1957 theory.

The analogy, in retrospect, was forced and offers little insight into the neural bases of language. But speculations along these lines continue. Davidson and Noble (1993) attempt to link the evolution of the modern human brain to the pace of technological innovation. They propose that the human brain reached its final form 50,000 years before the present (B.P.), ascribing the innovations of that time—bone needles, polished stone tools, ornaments, sculpture and paintings—to fully developed human cognitive and linguistic ability. However, neither material culture nor technology necessarily reflects a change in the brain. Oldowan tools were still being made and used in the closing years of the nineteenth century (Kingdon, 1993). If we were to link brain development with technology, we would have to conclude that a profound advance in human cognitive ability occurred between 1800 and the present.

Paul Mellars (1996), who has studied many Neanderthal sites, believes that many of the stone tools, ornaments, and objects found therein were borrowings from contemporary anatomically modern humans. Other late (about 34,000 years B.P.) Neanderthal sites also show signs of cultural borrowing between the last Neanderthals and the first modern humans in Europe (Hublin et al., 1996). Borrowing might imply that Neanderthals were incapable of devising these tools on their own. However, other archaeologists dispute this theory and claim that Neanderthal toolmaking was not influenced by contemporary *Homo sapiens* (D'Errico et al., 1998). In any event, it would be difficult to reach a definite conclusion concerning the cognitive and linguistic differences that might have existed between contemporary human populations and Neanderthals even if the Neanderthals had borrowed technology; although contemporary societies throughout the world today often borrow technology, that fact clearly does not signify any neural distinctions.

Some distinctions between Neanderthal and early human culture may have existed. Shea (1998) suggests that Neanderthal hunting practices and weapons differed from those of early modern humans. The early anatomically modern human Skhul V and Jabel Quafzeh fossils dated to about 100,000 years B.P., were found buried with "symbolic tools"—grave goods (McCowen and Keith, 1939; Vandermeersch, 1981). The connection may be significant; it would have been impossible to conceive of the need for grave goods without advanced linguistic-cognitive ability. Grave goods are not found in Neanderthal burial sites until much later periods; an example is the cave bear skulls associated with the La Ferassie Neanderthal burial site in France. The skeletal morphology of the basicranium of the Skhul V and Jabel Quafzeh fossils could have supported only a modern human SVT (Lieberman, 1975, 1984). These early modern humans therefore had the anatomical prerequisites for fully modern human speech and concomitant deficits in swallowing and chewing, as well as increased susceptibility to impacted teeth.[9] There would have been no reason for early modern humans to retain the odd human SVT unless they also possessed brains capable of regulating speech. Moreover, we can be certain that the human FLS existed 100,000 years ago, at the time of the migration of humans from Africa and their subsequent dispersal throughout most of the world over the next 50,000 years. Otherwise we would find differences in the linguistic capabilities of human children native to different parts of the world. This is not the case; any normal human child will acquire any human language if exposed to a normal environment in early childhood.

The Demise of the Neanderthals

Phonetic ability also may account for one of the puzzling facts concerning hominid evolution, the extinction of the Neanderthals. If we follow Darwin's principle of "uniformitarianism" and assume that our ancestors acted as we do, then we must consider the effects of distinctions in dialect in mate selection. Barbujani and Sokal (1990, 1991) have shown that dialects serve as a genetic isolating mechanism in present-day human populations. Using data from blood-grouping studies of European populations, they found that sharp genetic differences appeared along physical boundaries, such as mountain ranges or large bodies of water, that prevent people from intermingling. This was not surprising. However, they also found similar genetic discontinuities among different groups of people who could have intermingled but spoke different languages (Finnish versus Russian) or different dialects of Italian or German. Dialect distinctions appear to have genetically isolated human populations in the recent past for thousands of years, even though any child growing up in any linguistic environment will effortlessly acquire the native dialect. Dialect distinctions would have served to genetically isolate anatomically modern human and Neanderthal populations with even greater force. Classic Neanderthals, such as people resembling the La Chapelle-aux-Saints fossil, would have been inherently unable to produce the "modern human" dialect of any language that included [i]s or [u]s. The demographic model developed by Zubrow (1990) predicts that slight differences in biological fitness could have accounted for Neanderthal extinction if they had been genetically isolated from contemporary human populations over many generations. Thus, we can account for the fact that Neanderthals are extinct without invoking wars of extermination or radically superior cognitive or linguistic ability for anatomically modern humans.[10]

Qualitative Distinctions between Hominid and Ape Brains

One solution to why human beings have superior cognitive and linguistic abilities relative to living apes would be that our brains are qualitatively different. As noted, Chomsky proposed a language organ instantiating a Universal Grammar, but no such organ has been isolated in living human beings. Other neurobiological studies also have attempted to link human linguistic ability to a qualitative neural distinction. Geschwind and Levitsky (1968) claimed that the planum temporale (PT), a site within Wernicke's area, was the key to human language. Anatomical asymmetry was found in Wernicke's area and the PT; the left-hemisphere PT was much larger in human brains than in the right hemisphere of the brain. In contrast, Geschwind and Levitsky noted the absence of this asymmetry when they examined the brains of chimpanzees. Following the implicit principle that cortical left-hemisphere dominance is the key to human linguistic ability, they concluded that PT asymmetry was a qualitative neural distinction that explained human linguistic ability. However, Gannon et al. (1998) demonstrate that the chimpanzee PT shows the same asymmetry as occurs in humans. Gannon and his colleagues suggest alternate interpretations of their finding: either chimpanzees have the neural capacity for complex human language, or PT asymmetry is irrelevant to language. Other studies indicate that the latter is the correct interpretation. Galaburda et al. (1985) observed that some humans who have difficulty reading but possess language and speech have less asymmetric PTs than other humans. However, 67 percent of the perfectly normal individuals studied by Galaburda and his colleagues showed the putative asymmetry. If PT asymmetry were really the key to language, these subjects possessing symmetric PTs would have had profound linguistic deficits. Moreover, chimpanzees do not talk or possess the linguistic ability of humans who are slow readers. Reading is a recent innovation; most of the world's humans are still illiterate although they possess language. A reasonable conclusion is that PT asymmetry is irrelevant to language.

Deacon (1988, 1997) has suggested that the proportion of the prefrontal cortex relative to other parts of the human brain increased by 200 percent compared to apes. As previous chapters have noted, regions of the prefrontal cortex support neuronal populations that form part of the circuits implicated in abstract cognition, language, and speech. Deacon ascribes these human attributes to the disproportionate increase in the prefrontal cortex and links to the cerebellum. If we take into account the size of the human brain versus the brain size that we would expect for a given body size in a mammal, an "encephalization quotient" (EQ) can be calculated. An EQ of 1.0 would mean that brain size was proportional to the average body size across all mammals. The human brain shows a higher EQ than other primates', about 7.0 compared to 2.4 for chimpanzees (Jerison, 1973). However, it is not clear that this increase in brain size derives from a disproportionate increase of the frontal or prefrontal neocortex. Semendeferi et al. (1997) determined the volume of the frontal lobe of the neocortex relative to the entire brain in MRIs of living humans and in postmortem examinations of chimpanzees, gorillas, orangutans, gibbons, and macaques. The proportion of frontal lobe to brain size is similar in all hominoids. Moreover, the relative size of the dorsal, mesial, and orbital sectors of the frontal lobe is similar in all hominoids. These observations are consistent with the data of Stephan, Frahm, and Baron (1981), who used tightly controlled procedures to measure the volume of various parts of the brains of humans and other species. Data on more than 2,000 volumetric measurements of 42 brain structures for 76 species were reported. The total volume of the chimpanzee (*Pan troglodytes*) brain that they measured was 382,103 mm^3; the human brain's volume was 1,251,847 mm^3, 3.3 times larger. Compared to the chimpanzee brain, the human neocortex is only 3.45 times larger. Most human subcortical structures except the cerebellum showed proportionately smaller increases in volume: the striatum (caudate nucleus and putamen) is 2.34 times larger, the globus pallidus is 2.41 times greater, the thalamus is 2.45 times greater, and the cerebellum is 3.15 times larger.

The question is still not resolved, but the human neocortex and prefrontal cortex may not be disproportionately larger than would be expected from the general increase of the human brain's volume. However, an increase of computational power deriving from the overall larger size of the neocortex may account for the qualitatively different functional "power" of the human brain. Similar qualitative functional differences are evident when one considers the range of problems that can be solved using a 1960s-vintage digital computer and current supercomputers. Quantitative increases in memory and computational speed have yielded qualitative differences in computer "behavior." Complex programs that simply were impossible to implement thirty years ago routinely solve qualitatively different problems.

Bipedalism, Sign Language, and Early Hominid Language

The selective pressures that resulted in the evolution of human speech may ultimately derive from upright bipedal locomotion, the initial hominid adaptation. As noted earlier, the demands of bipedal locomotion may have selected for the evolution of enhanced subcortical motor control structures (basal ganglia and cerebellum) that regulate walking. Various theories have been proposed to account for the evolution of bipedal upright locomotion. However, upright posture clearly freed hominid hands. Virtually all aspects of human behavior would be affected if we could not use our hands to touch, hold, and manipulate whatever we chose. Further selection for manual dexterity and control may have occurred. Speech communication can be regarded as a biological extension of upright posture's freeing hominid hands for work. Although manual sign languages, which were invented about 200 years ago, can convey subtle linguistic distinctions (Stokoe, 1978), they limit this capability. Manual gestural language inherently places greater demands on its user when another manual task must be carried out. However, gestural communication is part of our daily life; it complements spoken language. Virtually everyone uses hand gestures to indicate movement and emphasize words. Certain gestures also supplement the acoustic cues that signal phrase and sentence boundaries and other linguistic information (McNeill, 1985). However, these gestures supplement speech; the full range of linguistic distinctions can be transmitted in a telephone conversation and to a somewhat lesser degree in a written form. Moreover, current neurobiological data show that the neural structures that process transient visual signals and the neural structures used to process speech in hearing persons work together to process manual sign language in hearing-impaired persons (Bellugi, Poizner, and Klima, 1983; Hickok, Bellugi, and Klima, 1996; Nishimura et al., 1999).[11] This is not surprising in light of other observations concerning the plasticity of the brain noted earlier. Touch was the medium that allowed Helen Keller to acquire language. But manual ability, speech, and language may be linked.

It is possible that the initial stages of hominid language relied to a greater extent on manual gestures (Hewes, 1973). Similar functions and morphology mark the striatal-cortical circuits implicated in manual motor control and cognitive behavior (Cummings, 1993; Marsden and Obeso, 1994), and a linkage between the neural mechanisms that regulate precise manual motor control and language has been suggested in previous studies (Lieberman, 1973, 1975, 1984, 1985, 1991; Kimura, 1979; MacNeilage, 1987). As noted earlier, deficits in manual motor control frequently are a consequence of brain damage that results in permanent aphasia.

The neural bases of manual sign language clearly are more primitive, since chimpanzees can master childlike ASL. And simple sign language can be mastered by some mentally retarded people (primarily severe Down's syndrome) who are not able to talk (Wills, 1973). Deaf children spontaneously invent primitive sign languages (Goldin-Meadow, 1993; Goldin-Meadow and Mylander, 1998). However, it is not clear that they have anything that might be characterized as grammar. Their communications appear to conform more closely to the mimetic theory proposed by Donald (1991) for the initial stages of human language than to the linguistic categorization proposed by Goldin-Meadow and Mylander. The neural bases for precise manual motor control are apparent in the increasingly complex stone tools that constitute much of the archaeological record of early hominid culture. Selection for enhanced voluntary manual motor control evidenced in the archaeological record would have allowed communication by means of manual sign language. At some point in hominid evolution circuits supporting voluntary speech evolved. The unanswered question is when.

Bound versus Adaptive Behavior

One line of research that might answer this question would involve determining what enables human beings to "unpack" the sequential elements that form "bound" responses to external stimuli, forming novel flexible motoric or cognitive outputs (Lieberman, 1994a). As noted in Chapter 4, recent studies indicate that circuits supported in a number of structures of the FLS (including striatum, globus pallidus, thalamus, anterior caudate nucleus, and prefrontal cortex) may be implicated in shifting cognitive sets, making inferences, forming abstractions, and so on. The studies reviewed earlier (e.g., Kimura, Aosaki, and Graybiel, 1993; Wise, 1997) show that the brains of animals besides humans have neural mechanisms that adapt to different learning experiences to produce timely motoric responses to environmental challenges and opportunities. Indeed such mechanisms can be found in very simple animals such as mollusks (Carew, Waters, and Kandel, 1981). The evolution of more complex brains, in part, appears to involve adaptations that increased biological fitness by allowing animals to adapt to changing environments through behavioral modifications, rather than by hardwired genetically transmitted "instincts." It is clear, for example, that dogs have more adaptable behavioral responses to a greater variety of situations than toads. In a meaningful sense, a functional neural system that is malleable, that "learns" to produce a rapid motoric response that enhances biological fitness to some range of "novel" situations, is a *cognitive* system. In response to the Darwinian "struggle for existence," functional neural systems evolved that are not bound to stereotyped responses to a limited range of environmental stimuli—responses "bound" to a situation or mental set.

The functions performed by the subcortical neural mechanisms of the FLS seem to reflect this evolutionary hierarchy. For example, in rodents the basal ganglia support circuits that regulate submovement sequencing of an innate grooming "program" (Berridge and Whitshaw, 1992; Aldridge et al., 1993). In contrast, in monkeys the basal ganglia circuits also appear to be formed as the submovements of complex motor activity are learned (Kimura, Aosaki, and Graybield, 1993; Graybiel et al., 1994). Similar arguments have been made for the formation of circuits involving the prefrontal cortex and cerebellum (Grafman, 1989; Grafman et al., 1992; Thatch et al., 1993; Goel and Grafman, 1995; Raymond, Lisberger, and Mauk, 1996). Vocal communication appears to be bound to affect in nonhuman primates (Pierce, 1985). It is clear that neural circuitry evolved that allowed hominids to produce voluntary speech, transcending the communicative limits of bound, stereotyped vocalizations. Since the neuroanatomical structures that regulate voluntary human speech also underlie the "abstract" thought processes that are exemplified in human linguistic ability, this might account for enhanced hominid cognitive and linguistic ability. But the question that presently eludes us is how these circuits were formed, if indeed any species-specific circuits occur in *Homo sapiens.*

Parrots and Other "Talking" Birds

One possible objection to one of the major premises of this book, that speech is a central aspect of human linguistic ability, might be the existence of "talking" birds. Parrots and other birds seemingly have the ability to talk. In fact Pepperberg (1981) showed that one parrot named Alex vocalized a limited number of words in a productive manner instead of merely "parroting" them. However, acoustic analyses of the vocalizations of mynah birds, parrots, and other passerines show that the signals that human listeners perceive as speechlike do not have characteristics of human speech (Greenewalt, 1968; Klatt and Stefanski, 1974). Whereas the phonetic information of human speech is conveyed by a complex pattern of formant frequency transitions imposed on laryngeal and noise sources, talking birds instead place almost "pure" sinusoidal tones on the points in the frequency spectrum that approximate the spectral peaks of the speech signal that correspond to formant frequencies. Passerines can generate these signals by means of their syringes, sound-producing structures that are derived features of birds. Similar effects can be produced by synthesizing speechlike stimuli with sinusoidal tones (Remez et al., 1981); listeners will accept these stimuli as speech signals when prompted to do so.[12] However, they easily differentiate these sounds from actual speech sounds. Similar effects occur when people listen to "talking" parrots, if the listener is prepared to accept the sound as speech. However, listeners readily differentiate parrot vocalizations from human speech.

Patterson and Pepperberg (1994) claim that the "vowels" produced by the parrot Alex are differentiated by means of formant frequency patterns. However, their published data suggest that the perceived phonetic distinctions were not produced by the parrot's changing the filter function of his airway. The parrot Alex would have had to be a rather large parrot having a vocal tract that was approximately 15 cm long in order to generate the claimed formant frequency patterns, which in any case do not include the vowels [i] and [u]. Moreover, the published vowel spectra (ibid., p. 638) do not show a fundamental frequency and harmonics modulated by the filter function of the SVT. No energy is apparent below the supposed second formant frequency of the vocalization that Patterson and Pepperberg perceived as the vowel [u]. But the issue of parrot speech is in a broader sense irrelevant to the evolution of human speech and language. The particular speech-producing anatomy and neural mechanisms regulating speech and language in human beings are the result of our particular evolutionary history. In a different universe, birds that had large brains might have evolved that could have used the different sound-producing anatomy and auditory system of birds to communicate a vocal language with the full power of human language. However, we are not descended from birds; the structures produced by the processes of biological evolution follow from its "proximate," historical logic (Mayr, 1952). Hence, though talking birds are interesting in themselves and may demonstrate the proposition that other species may communicate to a limited degree by means of symbolic systems that have some of the properties of human language, they do not refute the proposition that a functional language system in which speech plays a central role is one of the derived properties of *Homo sapiens*.

Concluding Comments

There seems to be no compelling reason to accept theories that propose discontinuities, that human language suddenly appeared full-blown from a "protolanguage" by means of a unique biological process (e.g., Bickerton, 1990), or theories that rely on unverifiable scenarios and a hypothetical "cheater-detector" (Bickerton, 1998b; Calvin and Bickerton, 2000). The Darwinian processes that appear to account for the evolution of communication in other species (Hauser, 1996) can account for the evolution of the proposed functional language system and many of its properties—the apparent linkages between neural mechanisms regulating speech, language, and cognition. Neural mechanisms that were initially adapted for one purpose, perhaps walking and manual motor control, took on "new" functions, speech motor control, the regulation of complex syntax, and certain aspects of cognition. Structures of the brain performing particular "computations," such as sequencing, fortuitously effected these operations in these "new" modes of behavior and subsequently were modified by means of natural selection. Natural selection acted to perfect these new neural functions, since language enhances virtually all aspects of human behavior that increase biological fitness. The roots of present human linguistic ability probably go back to our distant ape-human ancestor. Lexical ability and simple syntax probably were present from the start, speech soon afterward. Syntax is not the touchstone of human language. Syntactic ability undoubtedly was present in a limited degree in the earliest hominids. When speech or complex syntax came into being probably will never be known, but some of the necessary neural and anatomical prerequisites were present from the start of hominid evolution.

In short, the theory that Charles Darwin proposed can account for the evolution of the proposed functional language system.

CHAPTER 6

Commentary

Speech is a central, if not the central, feature of human linguistic ability. Although the human brain is plastic and can adapt to other input-output modes, vocal speech is the default condition. The function of the neural system, the FLS, that regulates human language is to rapidly transmit, comprehend, and store information, and to think using the medium of speech. Human speech achieves a high data-transmission rate, accesses words, and maintains words and their semantic, syntactic, and pragmatic referents in verbal working memory, where the "meaning" of a sentence is derived. And in our minds we can think in the words of inner speech.

It is evident that present-day humans have specialized brain mechanisms that allow us to talk, transmitting the conceptual information coded as words and integrating other information (visual, tactile, pragmatic) with the knowledge coded in the words of our internal lexicon. Words are powerful conceptual as well as communicative elements. The word *tree* doesn't necessarily refer to a particular tree or even to a species. *Tree* codes a concept. The conceptual information coded in the brain's lexicon appears to recruit information represented in structures of the brain concerned with sensation and motor control. For example, when we say or think of the word *pencil* we activate the shape and color information stored in the visual cortex (Martin et al., 1995). Therefore, linguistic knowledge is knowledge of the external world, stored within the brain in the form of words that are accessed through the sounds of human speech. And inner speech is a medium of human thought.

The functional language system that effects these processes is a distributed, parallel network. Neural circuits formed by populations of neurons in many neuroanatomical structures process and transmit signals to other neuronal populations. A given neuroanatomical structure can support neuronal populations that play a role in circuits that regulate other aspects of behavior in other functional neural systems. It is evident that subcortical neural structures that regulate other aspects of motor control support circuits of the FLS that regulate speech and also play a part in comprehending sentences. Subcortical basal ganglia structures also play a part in "abstract" cognition. The FLS contributes to biological fitness by rapidly integrating sensory information and conceptual information with prior knowledge, represented in the shape of words and sentences, to produce appropriate responses to the outside environment or internal mental states. In a sense, human language and thought can be regarded as neurally "computed" motor activity, deriving from neuroanatomical systems that generate overt motor responses to environmental challenges and opportunities. In short, the anatomy and physiology of the human FLS reflects its evolutionary history. Natural selection operated on motor control systems that provide timely responses to environmental challenges and opportunities.

Comparative studies show that although apes cannot talk, they have limited lexical and syntactic ability. And so we can conclude that the neural bases of lexical ability and syntax are primitive features that must have been present in early hominids. The derived properties of human language, speech and elaborated syntax, entail the evolution of the human FLS. Studies of the evolution of human speech anatomy provide some insights into the time course of the evolution of human language as well as the extinction of archaic hominid species. The nature of the adaptations that yielded human speech capability and enhanced human syntactic and cognitive ability remains unclear. But it is clear that the basal ganglia and other subcortical structures are essential elements of the FLS, supporting circuits implicated in speech, syntax, and some aspects of abstract cognition. Therefore, studies of the evolution of Broca's and Wernicke's areas of the neocortex, in themselves, cannot solve the riddle of human language and thought; we must also account for the evolution of the cortico-striatal circuits that regulate these human capacities.

Evolution and Cognitive Science

The evidence presented in this book indicates that the functional morphology of the human brain should be viewed in the light of evolution. The proximate, opportunistic logic of evolution has produced a brain in which subcortical structures that regulate motor control in phylogenetically primitive animals are key components of circuits that regulate human language and thought. Other comparative studies suggest that the homologue of Broca's area in nonhuman primates also regulates manual motor activity (Rizzolatti et al., 1996; Rizzolatti and Arbib, 1998). Cognitive scientists have attempted to understand mind-brain relations using modular theories that owe more to IBM than to Charles Darwin. However, the constraints of evolutionary biology that structure the anatomy and physiology of the human brain cannot be ignored. Cognitive science must take the principles and lessons of evolutionary biology into account.

Localization of Function

It is clear that the nineteenth-century model that equates Broca's and Wernicke's areas with the neural "seats" of human linguistic ability is wrong. However, the focus here on the subcortical basal ganglia must not be interpreted as a claim that either speech motor control or syntax resides in the basal ganglia. The FLS integrates activity in many parts of the human brain, including the subcortical cerebellum, thalamus, motor cortex, premotor cortex, prefrontal regions, and sensory cortex. The basal ganglia appear to sequence automatized motor programs represented in the neocortex. Basal ganglia also appear to sequence automatized syntactic processes, which probably have a cortical representation. The memory traces that constitute the many "meanings" of a word surely are represented cortically. However, imaging data suggest that the neural representation of the "meaning" of a word enlists the cortical regions that are activated in the perception of the colors, shapes, and other properties of the objects and actions coded in a word, such as the motor activity that may define a word through its function (e.g., hand movements for a hammer). In this light, the meaning of the sentence *The boy was running* reduces to an internal image of a boy running. The inference that follows is that, contrary to traditional, formal linguistic theory, predicate logic does not characterize the neural bases of human semantic knowledge.

Linguistic Algorithms

The evidence presented here also suggests that the algorithmic methods that characterize most formal linguistic studies are not appropriate tools if we wish to understand better the mind-brain relations that govern linguistic ability. More than forty years have passed since Noam Chomsky initiated linguistic studies directed at discovering the universals of human language. However, candid exponents of the algorithmic approach introduced by Chomsky such as Ray Jackendoff (1994, p. 26) admit they cannot even describe the sentences of any human language. Despite the sustained efforts by hundreds of trained linguists, only a small subset of the sentences of any language can be described by means of algorithmic, syntactic "rules." The sentences that can be characterized by means of algorithms conforming to successive, somewhat different versions of generative grammar of the Chomskian school typically are the examples presented in introductory courses. As the linguistic corpus expands, the number of algorithms also dramatically increases. The algorithms necessary to describe the expanded corpus become torturously complex and ultimately fail. In short, although many theoretical linguists claim that they have discovered the "universals" of human language, I doubt that the sentences in this chapter could be described using an algorithmic approach.

This failure clearly does not stem from stupidity, incompetence, or lack of motivation. The neurobiologic evidence discussed throughout this book suggests that linguists should consider a biologically motivated approach, characterizing the mental operations that human beings use to comprehend language by means of parallel, distributed processes similar to those that regulate motor control. As Darwin and virtually all subsequent evolutionary biologists have stressed, biological evolution is opportunistic; as I have repeatedly noted, the neuroanatomical organization of the FLS does not differ substantially from that of the functional neural systems regulating motor control. The "computations" carried out by basal ganglia structures do not appear to differ whether syntax or finger motions are the distal goals. Keeping this in mind, linguists should note that these computations are not algorithmic. One of the threads that unite many studies of motor control is that the neural "instruction sets" that guide particular motor acts are not equivalent in shape or form to algorithms. On the basis of the motor system's known basal ganglia and cortical anatomy and physiology, Alexander, Delong, and Crutcher, three distinguished specialists on the neural bases of motor control, conclude:

> The general concept that the motor system uses computational algorithms to control movements, as well as the more specific notion that motor programs are involved, began to become popular at a time when relatively little

> was known about the structural and functional organization of the motor system . . . However, with the progressive refinement of our knowledge of the motor system's anatomy and physiology, the motor programming concept has become increasingly divorced from any apparent relevance to the neural substrates of motor control.
>
> Instead we suggest that the motor system, including (but not limited to) the extended network comprising the cortical and basal ganglionic motor areas, is more likely to process information through a process that is essentially "nonalgorithmic," one that depends on a characteristically biological form of neural architecture that is at once self-organizing, highly parallel, and massively interconnected. (1992, pp. 656–657)

Given the similar structure and physiology of the cortical–basal ganglia components of neural motor control systems and the FLS, a nonalgorithmic approach to characterizing human knowledge of syntax might merit consideration by theoretical linguists. Algorithmic descriptions of linguistic phenomena are perfectly valid tools so long as they are not equated with the mental operations carried out by the human brain. And linguists should continue to study the varied syntactic and semantic characteristics of the languages of the world. But time and effort have been wasted in the linguistic quest to discover the "true" set of algorithms that describe linguistic "competence," the fund of linguistic knowledge coded by the human brain. The effort is inherently misdirected because the brain's neural computations do not, in any sense, correspond to serial, algorithmic processes.

Learning Language

A second lesson can be drawn from studies of the neural bases of motor control. Robust data from many independent studies show that neural circuits involving cortical and subcortical structures are formed as animals or humans learn to perform particular motor tasks. Neural plasticity is a general phenomenon (e.g., Merzenich et al., 1984; Merzenich, 1987; Sanes and Donoghue, 1996, 1997, in press; Donoghue, 1995; Karni et al., 1995, 1998; Pascual-Leone et al., 1995; Sanes and et al., 1995; Elman et al., 1996; Nudo et al., 1996; Classen et al., 1998). The particular neural circuits that regulate many complex aspects of human and animal behavior are shaped by exposure to an individual's environment during these sensitive periods.

Neural plasticity marks perception as well as motor control. Edelman's

(1987) review of the data of hundreds of studies points out a metaphorical "struggle for existence" in which neuronal pathways that are not used deteriorate. Neuroanatomical experiments, for example, show that inputs to the visual cortex develop in early life in accordance with visual input; different visual inputs yield different input connections (Hata and Stryker, 1994). In fact, cortical regions that normally respond to visual stimuli in cats instead respond to auditory and tactile stimuli in visually deprived cats. Rauschecker and Korte (1993) monitored single-neuron activity in the anterior visual cortical area of normal cats and cats that had been vision deprived. Neurons in this area in normal cats had purely visual responses. In young cats who had been deprived of vision from birth only a minority of cells in this area responded to visual stimuli, but most responded vigorously to auditory and to some extent somatosensory stimuli.[1] Similar phenomena have now been found to characterize brain-language relationships. Nisimura et al. (1999) show that the secondary auditory cortex responds to the gestures of manual sign language in deaf people. And virtually all linguists note that a "critical" or "sensitive" period exists in which children effortlessly acquire the ability both to perform the motor acts necessary to speak a dialect with a "native" accent and to master syntax and morphology. Thus, it is difficult to see how linguists can argue for a special innate Universal Grammar that structures the acquisition of linguistic knowledge.

Associative Learning

Many linguists and philosophers also short-change the power of associative learning. For example, the categorical perception of syllable-onset formant patterns by human infants (Eimas, 1974) has generally been taken as one of the strongest demonstrations that human beings have innate specialized devices, "feature detectors" tuned to the specific characteristics of speech (Lieberman, 1975, 1984; Pinker, 1994).[2] However, a comparatively simple simulation of an associative neural network modeled on current knowledge of neocortical physiology can "learn" to identify the formant frequency patterns that specify stop consonants in syllables such as [ba], [da] and [ga] (Seebach et al., 1994). Seebach's study shows that innate knowledge is not necessary; the computer-implemented simulation correctly identified these sounds in a categorical manner after a limited number of trials.[3] Human infants clearly have associative powers that transcend those of the simple neural network used by Seebach; human infants also are exposed to hundreds of hours of speech, which they can hear in the last month of gestation prior to birth. Hence we need assume no innate knowledge of the particular characteristics of human speech to account for the observed categorical identification of stop consonants by human infants.

Rumelhart and McClelland (1986) showed that a simple neural network model could "acquire" and then overgeneralize one aspect of English verb morphology in stages that are very similar to those in young children. The point of this study was that this process could be accomplished with an exceedingly *simple* network. The objections to Rumelhart and McClelland's model raised by Pinker and Prince (1988) missed this point. Later network simulations (MacWhinney, 1991) addressed some of the specific points raised by Pinker and Prince; Churchland (1995) presents the results and discusses the implications of recent neural net simulations. But the real lesson, that neural nets that have extremely limited computational resources compared to the brain of even a mouse, can "acquire" rule-governed knowledge of language, that is, "linguistic competence," has eluded many theoretical linguists and cognitive scientists. This fact has been evident for many years; F. Liberman's (1979) extremely simple neural net simulation deduced the "rules" of a "matrix grammar," equivalent in generative power to the "transformational" grammars of that period.[4] Although no associative distributed neural net has yet mastered the syntax of any language, neither have linguists been able to describe the syntax of any human language (Jackendoff, 1994).

Current data (e.g., Singleton and Newport, 1989) are consistent with the idea that children learn syntax by means of associative learning (imperfectly modeled in simulated neural networks). In contrast to most developmental studies of language acquisition, the language input to the deaf child studied by Singleton and Newport was known, being limited to the American Sign Language produced by his deaf parents, who were imperfect signers. Whereas the child's parents, who were the models for the child, made errors 40 percent of the time for certain ASL signs, the child had a 20 percent error rate. These data have been interpreted as evidence for Universal Grammar. Pinker (1994, pp. 38–39), for example, claims that this demonstrates that the child had innate knowledge of the principles underlying ASL; otherwise he could not have performed better than his parents. What Pinker fails to note is that the child had a higher error rate than his parents when they incorrectly modeled other ASL signs more than 50 percent of the time. Therefore, the complete Singleton and Newport data set refutes Pinker's claim; the child's behavior is instead consistent with his deriving a "prototype" by means of associative mechanisms. This finding should not be surprising; pigeons can derive abstract "prototypes" through repeated exposure to many specific examples, enabling them to categorize different species of trees or tropical fish (Herrnstein, 1979; Herrnstein and De Villiers, 1980).

The degree of convergence and divergence in cortical–basal ganglia neural circuitry and the observed plasticity of the cortex appear to provide the necessary computational architecture for neural networks capable of associative learning. Alexander, Delong, and Crutcher again concur, noting that "much of the gross topography/somatotopy within the motor system may be genetically determined, whereas the fine-tuning . . . may depend significantly upon experience and associated activity-dependent changes in local synaptic weights" (1992, p. 661).[5]

Universal Grammar

Apart from the cogent arguments raised by Jeffrey Elman and his colleagues (1996) concerning neural plasticity (discussed in Chapter 3), these facts argue against Noam Chomsky's major biologic claim for a Universal Grammar (UG), the hypothetical set of innate "principles and parameters" that supposedly is a characteristic of all "normal" human brains. The UG specifies the total range of morphologic and syntactic rules that can exist in any language. According to linguists who share Chomsky's views, children do not learn the rules that govern syntax by means of general cognitive processes. The principles and parameters coded in the Universal Grammar instead are activated to yield the correct grammar of a particular language as a child is exposed to his or her linguistic environment. The burden of proof rests on linguists who claim that the circuits that code the details of language are innately determined, given the body of evidence that demonstrates that the details of motor control and many aspects of perception are not genetically determined. No evidence exists that suggests that the neural machinery regulating language differs fundamentally from that regulating other aspects of behavior.

Genetic Variation

It is also apparent that the basic facts on which evolutionary biology rests place a further burden of proof on linguists who claim that a Universal Grammar exists. The precise form of the UG has changed with Chomsky's different theories of syntax. However, the central biological claim preserved in all these formulations is that the UG is genetically transmitted. One of the keystones of the theory that Charles Darwin proposed in 1859 and that has been supported by all subsequent research is the universal presence of genetic variation. About 150 years of systematic investigation shows that genetic variation is, as Darwin claimed, a characteristic of all organisms. There is at least 10 percent variation in the alleles at any chromosome site in mammals (Mayr, 1982). The genetic makeup of virtually all living organisms, except for identical twins, clones, and the like, varies to some degree. This is apparent in the varying physical appearance of the individual members of any species. The effects of genetic variation are apparent when various aspects of behavior are studied. Color "blindness" and color deficiencies, for example, occur in human beings as a result of defective genes that code the innate color receptors of the primate visual system. Since the color receptors are discretely coded, other aspects of vision are generally spared in people afflicted by defective color vision. If the Universal Grammar really existed, we would expect to find some individuals who were unable to comprehend some fragment of the grammar of their native language because they lacked a specific "grammar gene." However, the supposed evidence for such behavior, the claimed linguistic deficits of family KE offered by Gopnick and her associates (Gopnik, 1990; Gopnik and Crago, 1991) is false. General deficits in the acquisition of syntax and speech do occur in family KE (Varga-Khadem et al., 1995, 1998) and may occur in other individuals (Leonard, 1998), but deficits limited to specific fragments of grammar have never been documented.[6] Moreover, many instances of language deficits can be traced to more general deficiencies in auditory perception (Tallal, 1976), or, in the case of family KE, to impaired basal ganglia–cortical circuits (Vargha-Khadem et al., 1998).

Again, the message from biology is that linguistic research should be directed toward discovering and describing the phenomena that actually characterize human languages, rather than a search for universals that apply to restricted "core" grammars. As Massimo Piattelli-Palmarini, one of Chomsky's prominent advocates, once declared, the Chomskian linguistic movement is a worldwide religion.[7] The search for the Universal Grammar is perhaps best regarded as a search for a holy grail.

Evaluating Linguistic Theories in the Light of Biology

Finally, scientific theories must be tested. As is the case for other disciplines, theoretical linguists must take into account the degree to which a particular theory describes the sentences of a corpus. However, it is usually the case that different sets of algorithms can describe a given set of sentences. In that event linguists usually appeal to vague notions of "simplicity," "economy," or formal "elegance." In the short forty-year history of Chomskian linguistic analysis, entire frames of reference have been replaced by appeals to these vague "formal" criteria (the most recent sea-change being Chomsky's [1995] "minimalist" movement).

However, these criteria are irrelevant, since the stated ultimate goal of the linguistic enterprise is biological—to characterize the Universal Grammar that enables a child to acquire speech and language. The general principle that governs the logic of biology is that it is not logical. Ernst Mayr (1982) forcefully drives the point home: "proximate," historical logic characterizes biology. Evolution is a tinkerer, adapting existing structures that enhance reproductive success in the ever-changing conditions of life. There is no "logical" reason for supposing that the structures of the mammalian middle ear that enhance auditory sensitivity would have evolved from bones that hinge reptilian jaws. It happened by chance. Likewise, there is no logical reason why neural structures that control locomotion in human beings also play a part in thinking. Evolution does not give a damn about formal elegance.

Public Policy and the Study of Language

In many species instinct governs central aspects of behavior that are established with only limited exposure to appropriate stimuli. For example, ducks acquire their species-specific vocal calls after hearing these sounds while they are still hatchlings (Gottlieb, 1975). If language were an instinct, then only minimal attention would have to be paid to the circumstances in which children are raised. In this light, spending public funds to enrich the lives of children born into poverty would be unnecessary. Indeed, given the relationship that surely holds between language and cognition, we might conclude that the cognitive distinctions that some claim exist in various social, ethnic, and racial groups are fixed genetic properties. But even Herrnstein and Murray (1994), who claim to have documented these differences, note that environment shapes cognition. As the evidence discussed in this book demonstrates, language is a skill. Like other skills, such as playing the violin, certain neural and anatomical mechanisms are required. But like other skills, language is honed by practice in places and circumstances conducive to learning. The message here is that we as a nation have not done enough.

Brain, Language, and Thought

In closing the circle, it is appropriate to note that many questions posed in these chapters remain unanswered. It is clear that the functional organization of the human brain conforms to neither locationist, neophrenological, nor modular theories of the form postulated by many cognitive scientists. However, the degree to which neural circuits are segregated and committed to particular linguistic or other functions is uncertain. The default substrate for speech and language appears to be genetically determined, but it is clear that other neural structures can be enlisted when these "primary" structures are damaged. However, although some general constraints are apparent (e.g., extensive bilateral damage to the basal ganglia results in permanent loss of language), the limits on neural plasticity are unknown. The detailed circuitry of the FLS is an open question, as are the total effects of experience on circuit formation. And we do not know what really differentiates the human brain from that of an ape. Many, many detailed questions are unresolved, and when resolved will open further questions. But these questions can and will be addressed as imaging, tracer, and genetic-manipulative techniques progress. A better understanding of the neural bases of speech, language, and thought is a certainty.

Yet many linguists will feel that the answers to these biological issues are irrelevant to their interests, supposedly being outside the proper domain of linguistics. This view is apparent in the current hermetic isolation of formal linguistic research. Thus, the final message of this book is a call for biological linguistics, linguistic research that follows the model furnished by biology. Real science relates phenomena that previously appeared to be unrelated and explains those relationships. Understanding the nature of the human brain's functional language system will ultimately lead to understanding of the nature of human language and thought.

Notes

Introduction

1. Although Chomsky (personal communication) vehemently denies that he claimed that the neural bases of human language could not have evolved (1976, 1980b), he in effect claimed that human language could *not* have evolved by means of Darwinian processes. But Darwin's evolutionary theory is, as Mayr (1982) demonstrated, still the only game in town, so Chomsky's claims reduce to a belief in some unspecified unique biological process or other event that applied to human beings alone—human Cartesian uniqueness (Chomsky, 1966). Whether Chomsky still claims that human language (really syntax) could not have evolved by means of Darwinian processes is unclear.
2. The argument that formal, written text rather than actual conversation is the true embodiment of linguistic competence ignores the fact that writing is a recent invention in the context of human evolution. All but a small fraction of the world's population was illiterate until the twentieth century, millions of people are still illiterate, and children are generally illiterate in the period in which they acquire language.

1. Functional Neural Systems

1. Percheron and his colleagues (Percheron, Yelnick, and Francois, 1984; Percheron and Fillon, 1991), noting the extensive dendritic arborization in the basal ganglia, argue against completely segregated circuits. I return to this issue in Chapter 4.
2. The second place may be held by the view that the two hemispheres of the human brain work completely independently: the left hemisphere of the human brain supposedly regulates abstract thought and language; the right, art and emotion. So we are urged to draw using the right side of our brain.
3. Anderson (1995) presents a clear introduction to neural networks.

2. Speech Production and Perception

1. Other acoustic cues that play a part in VOT distinctions, such as greater release-burst amplitudes for [p]s, also derive from physiologic effects. The longer VOT of [p] compared to [b] means that the laryngeal opening is larger when a speaker's lips open at the release of the stop, yielding a higher airflow and consequent burst amplitude (Lieberman and Blumstein, 1988).
2. The formant frequencies of the vowel [i] also serve as an acoustic clue to the body size of a human speaker. Fitch (1994) presented synthesized [i]s and other vowels to listeners who were asked to judge the probable size of the speaker. Judgments based on [i] were most significantly correlated with body size. Fitch (1997) shows that in the rhesus macaque the formant structure of an animal's pant threats is highly correlated with its body size ($r = -0.771$, $p < 0.0002$). The high correlation for rhesus macaque follows from the fact that body size and vocal tract length are also highly correlated in this species ($r = 0.947$, $p < 0.0001$). Fitch proposes that neural mechanisms that relate formant frequencies to size have a communicative role in other animals, providing a preadaptive basis for vocal tract normalization in human speech. We will return to this issue in the final chapter.
3. Liberman and Mattingley (1985) and other studies (e.g., Pinker, 1994) assume that these categorical effects, which can be observed in infants, reflect innate knowledge that is part of a "speech module." However, as the next chapter notes, it is just as likely that they are learned early in life.
4. The phonetic details appear to include the different airflows that characterize different speech sounds (vowels use little air, fricatives more). You can observe this phenomenon by noting how you can "run out of air" when you utter a sentence that has high airflow demands such as "Henry hopped home."

3. The Lexicon and Working Memory

1. Damasio et al. (1996) interpret the mapping between phonological shape (the word's sound pattern) and meaning to a set of hierarchical semantic "features." The word *cat* would hypothetically be represented by a semantic feature tree that started with animate versus nonanimate, branched to animals versus humans, domestic animals versus wild animals, and perhaps a "level" in which "furry" versus "nonfurry" animals were specified. However, the experimental data could just as well reflect the categorization of animals versus humans by means of fuzzy prototypes similar to those formed by neural nets (Anderson, 1995) and the activity of the neural structures implicated in real-world use or perception coded by these words.
2. Ojemann et al. (1989) in a cortical stimulation study of 117 subjects found considerable intersubject variation in the locations of sites at which stimulation produced word-finding difficulties in an object-naming task. The sites included pos-

terior regions well outside the traditional language areas, including the sites noted by Damasio et al. (1996).

3. The possibility that the similarities that exist among languages derive from cultural transmission cannot be ruled out. Since Darwinian theory posits common ancestry for all living organisms, there must have been common ancestors for all modern human beings. "Eve" and "Adam" spoke some particular language, though we cannot easily "reconstruct" it. The "core" grammar hypothesized by Chomskian linguistics may reflect some properties of that ancestral language, modified in the course of time. The linguistic evidence favors monogenesis—a common language of which traces can be seen in the vocabularies of current languages (Ruhlen, 1994).
4. Longoni, Richardson, and Aiello (1993) dispute the decay of the phonologic representation of verbal material postulated by Baddeley and his colleagues. Longoni et al. tested the claim that performance in serial recall of verbal material involved both articulatory refreshment and short-term phonological coding. Serial recall is affected by word length; the number of long words that can be recalled is fewer than the number of short words for a given individual; this phenomenon presumably reflects the span of articulatory rehearsal. When subjects "suppress" articulatory rehearsal by speaking extraneous words during the recall test, their performance dramatically deteriorates, and the word-length effect disappears. Phonetically similar words are also more difficult to recall; articulatory suppression again dramatically decreases performance, but phonetic similarity in itself still results in an additional deterioration in recall. A 10-second delay between the presentation of the material that was to be remembered improved performance. Interference with articulatory rehearsal during the delay period yielded about the same reduction in recall for phonetically similar and dissimilar words. Longoni et al. interpret this result as indicating that the phonologic representation of a word is established immediately as it is heard and does not decay. In their view, the effects of suppressing articulatory rehearsal result from "overwriting" the phonologic representation. However, their theory does not account for the robust word-length effect that they replicate. A view consistent with Baddeley (1986) and the independent experimental data of Miles, Jones, and Madden (1991), involving delays in recall, is that the memory traces are strengthened by articulatory refreshment during the delay period.
5. According to Caplan, in a small portion of Broca's area (Stromswold et al., 1996). The localization is dubious; the PET averaging procedure used implicitly claims that the topographical organization of the cortex in different individuals is essentially identical. This is not the case (Ziles, 1995; Fink et al, 1997).
6. Aged normal subjects who may have reduced working memory spans also produce simplified syntax over the course of many years. Some aged people also have difficulty comprehending sentences that have complex syntax (Lieberman et al., 1989; Kemper, 1992; Bates et al., 1995). I will discuss this issue and the comprehension of syntax by agrammatic aphasics in relation to working memory in the next chapter.

7. In Stromswold et al. (1996) Caplan and the other coauthors note that they used a "pure" linguistic task, a grammaticality judgment that supposedly taps linguistic "competence." However, the different activation patterns that they find for right-branching versus center-embedded sentences must reflect "performance," since there is no theoretical difference between the complexity of the representation of either type of sentence. Stromswold and her colleagues, moreover, replicate the common finding that it takes more time to process a center-embedded sentence, whether the task is a picture-matching test of meaning or grammaticality judgment (Bates et al., 1992). Syntactic relations arguably code functional relations (Bates and MacWhinney, 1989; Croft, 1991).

4. The Subcortical Basal Ganglia

1. Brains perhaps cannot reroute the flow of information normally carried by subcortical circuits.
2. The presumed circuitry of the basal ganglia is complex and includes a "direct" path from the striatum to the internal segment of the globus pallidus (GPi) as well as an "indirect" pathway through the subthalamic nucleus and the external segment of globus pallidus (GPe). However, it is clear that the model is incomplete. Although the current model accounts for many observations, it fails to account for experimental data derived from studies of nonhuman primates and the results of surgery directed at ameliorating neurological impairments of humans (Delong, 1993; Marsden and Obeso, 1994).
3. Graybiel et al. (1994, p. 1827) note: "The estimated amount of divergence and convergence is impressive. The modules labelled from a roughly 1-mm-wide site in the sensorimotor cortex stretch over as much as 7 mm of the length and width of the putamen and fill a volume three to five times the volume of the cortical site from which they were labelled. The striatal modules labelled from a given site in the palladium [GP] have about the same dimensions."
4. Although neurologically intact subjects made very few grammaticality judgment errors in these experiments, the agrammatic aphasics had 20–30 percent error rates. Linebarger, Schwartz, and Saffran (1983) and Shankweiler et al. (1986) claimed that the impaired comprehension of distinctions of meaning in tests of sentence comprehension reflect semantic rather than syntactic deficits. However, error rates are always much higher in the absence of semantic constraints that would aid comprehension. Baum (1988) compared the performance of anterior aphasic subjects in an "on-line" lexical decision test and in grammaticality tests. She found that their performance was impaired in both types of tests and reflected difficulties in processing syntactic and/or morphological information.

   The focus on grammaticality judgments by linguists perhaps reflects the fact that linguistic studies generally fail to take into account experimental data reflecting comprehension. The "database" of theoretical linguistics often consists of introspective judgments of grammaticality made by the theoreticians themselves that sometimes result in bizarre, ostensibly "grammatical" sentences that exemplify "crucial" aspects of the theory of the moment.

5. Broca's aphasics and Parkinson's disease patients differ in this respect from persons suffering from dementia of Alzheimer's type who cannot associate a word with its semantic attributes. They, for example, won't remember the function of a *key*. Anomic Broca's subjects may not be able to recall the name *key* when presented with a key, but they are fully aware of its function.
6. Goldstein (1948) discusses several early studies of aphasia that noted lexical deficits restricted to proper names, animals, specific objects, similar to those described by Damasio et al. (1996).
7. The data of Natsopoulos et al. (1994) replicate the results of Lieberman, Friedman, and Feldman (1990) and Lieberman et al. (1992) insofar as higher error rates occurred when PD subjects were asked to comprehend sentences that had more-complex syntax. Their PD subjects, like those tested by Lieberman and colleagues and by Grossman et al. (1991, 1993), also made fewer errors when semantic information constrained the meaning of a sentence. For example, the fact that apples do not eat boys constrains the meaning of the sentence *The apple was eaten by the boy.* Although Natsopoulos and colleagues did not run any tests of cognition, they claim that no correlation exists between the comprehension of syntax and any other aspect of cognitive ability. Their claim is true if "linguistic" knowledge is equated with syntax—a position that seems implicit in many current linguistic studies.
8. ANOVAS showed that the VOT overlap subjects had significantly higher syntax error rates and longer response times on the RITLS than the VOT nonoverlap subjects—$F(1,70) = 12.38, p < 0.0008$; $F(1,70) = 7.70, p < 0.007$, respectively. The correlation between VOT timing errors and the number of syntax errors was $= 0.6473, p < 0.01$.
9. Differences in semantic priming occur for Broca's and Wernicke's syndromes. Broca's aphasics show normal priming effects when words are presented in pairs, but not over long time spans (Milberg, Blumstein, and Dworetzky, 1987, 1988). The pattern of semantic priming for Wernicke's aphasia is quite different. Wernicke's subjects show "hyperpriming" effects when compared with normal controls in similar tasks. They also show "spreading" phonetic priming effects, priming on words that are more phonetically dissimilar than is the case for normal control subjects. Milberg and colleagues ascribe these semantic priming effects to a reduction in lexical activation levels in Broca's aphasics and to a failure to inhibit lexical activation in the semantic network that constitutes long-term memory in Wernicke's aphasics. Although these effects may involve long-term memory, the phenomena noted in their experiments may instead involve working memory, since if a word cannot be maintained in working memory, it cannot be accessed from whatever neural substrate serves long-term memory. Phonetic information is maintained in working memory by "rehearsal." Therefore, the deterioration of speech motor sequencing of Broca's aphasics would reduce

their ability to "rehearse" words in working memory, necessarily resulting in less priming as working memory load increases over longer time spans. In contrast, the neuroanatomical structures that regulate speech production are spared in Wernicke's aphasia. The lexicon instead appears to be hyperactive, yielding multiple semantic outputs, disrupting comprehension.

Although semantic priming data for PD subjects are currently not available, the performance of PD subjects on naming tests suggests a lexical access deficit similar to that noted for Broca's aphasia. Verbal fluency as measured by initial-letter and semantic category retrieval has been extensively studied in PD. A typical initial-letter retrieval test involves a subject's producing as many words as possible, excluding proper names that begin with the letter *c* within 60 seconds, for example, *cat, canoe, canvas.* Although PD subjects who show relatively high deficits on other cognitive tests produce fewer words than normal controls, many nondemented PD subjects do not differ from controls. In contrast, deficits in naming within a semantic category, where subjects, for example, have to name as many animals as possible within 60 seconds, are frequently noted in studies of PD (Cohen et al., 1994). This difference in task difficulty contrasts with that of neurologically intact subjects, who generally find the semantic task easier, naming more words. The relative difficulty that PD subjects may have in lexical retrieval within a semantic category may reflect a working memory problem that results in deficits in lexical retrieval similar to those noted by Milberg, Blumstein, and Dworetzky (1987, 1988) for Broca's aphasics. Lexical retrieval involves maintaining the *name* of the semantic category in working memory throughout the task. Therefore, performance in the semantic category task would be impaired for those PD subjects having impaired speech motor control with concomitant impaired phonetic rehearsal. In contrast, the initial letter task imposes a lesser working-memory load, since each word furnishes the phonetic target for the next word.

10. Co-occurrence of VOT timing and sentence-comprehension deficits occurred on Chinese adaptations of the RITLS. Sentence-comprehension errors were significantly higher for sixteen of the PD subjects.
11. The aperiodic phonation that frequently occurs in Broca's aphasia as well as the "hypophonia" of PD may reflect damage to the neural circuitry regulating laryngeal activity. However, damage to this circuitry cannot explain VOT sequencing deficits. Impaired laryngeal function could perhaps explain why short VOTs for [b], [d], and [g] might be lengthened, but cannot explain why long VOTs for [p], [t], and [k] would be shortened.
12. The correlation coefficient was −0.774, $p < 0.001$. In contrast, performance was not impaired on cognitive tests involving the retrieval of words from memory, number spans forward and backward, and various tests of reasoning, including the Odd-Man-Out test (Flowers and Robertson, 1985). The possible effects of extreme cold and fatigue were ruled out; subjects were either in warm sunny conditions or were protected by tents and down clothing when they took these tests; their performance when they were most fatigued, after descending to Base

Camp shortly after reaching Everest's summit, was significantly better than at Camp Two or Three.

13. The imaging studies discussed in Chapter 3 (Awh et al., 1996; Just et al., 1996; Stromswold et al., 1996) suggest that Brodmann's area 45, which is usually considered to be part of Broca's area, is a key component of verbal working memory.
14. Disruptions in a person's ability to change cognitive criteria, thereby affecting the comprehension of distinctions in meaning conveyed by syntax in languages such as English or Chinese, which depend to a great degree on word order, would also apply to inflected languages such as Hindi, Greek, or Russian, in which similar distinctions are signaled by morphemes. The "decoding" process would have to involve switching from the information conveyed by a morpheme to that conveyed by the word stem. Disruptions in the production and comprehension of syntax occur in aphasia and Parkinson's disease in inflected languages (Bates, Frederici, and Wulfeck, 1987; Slobin, 1991; Wulfeck and Bates, 1991; Wulfeck, Bates, and Capasso, 1991; Bates and MacWhinney, 1989; Natsopoulos et al., 1994).
15. Studies of the ontogenetic development of human infants (Greenfield, 1991) also suggest that motor development and syntactic ability are linked. However, studies employing quantitative measures of both speech production and the comprehension of syntax are still lacking.

5. The Evolution of the Functional Language System

1. It is not surprising that the principles of evolutionary psychology have been endorsed by linguists following in Noam Chomsky's footsteps. Evolutionary psychology posits a specific genetic basis for virtually all aspects of human behavior. For example, Steven Pinker in a BBC interview ("The World," April 1998) stated that human beings are genetically predisposed to prefer landscapes that portray open vistas filled with greenery. Pinker asserts that we prefer these landscapes to heavily forested regions, mountains, deserts, seascapes, etc. We are informed that this preference is innate, deriving from genes shaped during the Pleistocene. According to Pinker these vistas of open greenery portray the open savannas of southern Africa where hominids first evolved. A visit to any major museum will refute this proposition; consider the highly valued classic Chinese paintings of travelers in the mountains, Turner's seascapes, Ansel Adam's mountain views, Edward Weston's desert scenes, and so on. Pinker is apparently unaware of recent archaeological studies that show that Australopithecine fossils and stone tools dated to the same epoch are found in parts of Africa that were heavily forested (White, Suwu, and Asfaw, 1994).

   But Pinker's scenario and corresponding aesthetic claims could readily be changed to account for these facts; Pinker could with equal certainty claim that we like to view these scenes because they portray the landscapes that our ancestors traversed as they migrated within and from Africa in past ages. In truth, the scenarios constructed by evolutionary psychologists are fables and are constructed to justify a genetic basis for any aspect of human behavior. It is not surprising that linguists working in the Chomskian tradition accept the premises of evolutionary psychology, since it generalizes Noam Chomsky's nativist agenda.

2. I have discussed the flawed conclusions of Terrace et al. (1979) elsewhere (Lieberman, 1984, 1991, 1998). Many studies cite Terrace's work as evidence that apes do not command any aspect of human language. The limits of Nim's (the chimpanzee trained by Terrace and his colleagues) linguistic ability reflect the deficiencies of the procedures used in their study.
3. The ice-age scenario ignores the fact that Europe was covered by 100 meters of ice during glacial maxima. Clearly, no hominids were resident during these periods.
4. The same point is stressed in Lieberman (1984, pp. 322–323).
5. Neanderthal speech capabilities are not the focus of this book. In fact, even if the Neanderthal SVT were capable of producing the full range of human speech sounds we would still have to address the question of when the human SVT evolved. Since the base of the skull is almost identical in chimpanzees and Australopithecine-grade hominids, there is no question that they had nonhuman SVTs (Lieberman, 1975, 1984; Laitman, Heimbuch, and Crelin, 1979; Laitman and Heimbuch, 1982). Therefore, at some point in hominid evolution an SVT adapted to enhance speech production and perception evolved. The Neanderthal speech debate has focused on the position of the larynx with respect to the base of the skull. The position of the larynx determines the length of the pharynx of the reconstruction of a fossil SVT. Edmund Crelin placed the Neanderthal larynx close to the base of its skull following the general principles of comparative anatomy. In closely related species, similar relationships generally hold between skeletal morphology and soft tissue. Therefore, since both metrical and qualitative assessments show that the skeletal features of the base of the skull that support the soft tissue of the SVT are similar in the La Chapelle-aux-Saints Neanderthal fossil and human newborns, it was reasonable to conclude that the SVTs were also quite similar.

   The polar opposites of the larynx-position debate are Crelin's reconstruction, in which the larynx is close to the base of the skull in a position similar to that of a human newborn's, and the Kebara Neanderthal reconstruction of Arensburg et al. (1990), who claim that its larynx occupied the same position as it does in an adult modern human, low in the neck. Unfortunately, Arensburg and his colleagues based their reconstruction on a fabricated scholarly reference to support the false assertion that the human larynx and the hyoid bone (a bone that supports the larynx) retain a fixed position in humans with respect to the cervical vertebrae and skull from birth onward. Arensburg and his colleagues, noting similarities between the shape of the Kebara Neanderthal fossil hyoid bone and human hyoid bones, argued that the Neanderthal hyoid and larynx must have occupied the low position that occurs in adult humans. All known anatomical data refute the Arensburg et al. argument. The human hyoid bone and larynx do not maintain a fixed position throughout life; they descend from high apelike position in the human neonate to a low position in normal adults (Negus, 1949; D. Lieberman and McCarthy, 1999). Furthermore, the human hyoid bone's shape doesn't change as it and the larynx descend. Therefore, the shape of the Kebara hyoid won't tell you where the Kebara Neanderthal's larynx was positioned (Lieberman, 1994b). The hyoid bone's shape is in fact irrelevant to the question of vocal anatomy. The hyoid bones of pigs and humans cannot be differentiated by the statistical metrics used by Arensburg et al., but pigs lack human speech-producing anatomy; the pig larynx, like the larynges of all quadrupeds, is positioned close to its skull.

Kay et al. (1998) attempt to assess the speech capabilities of Neanderthals by studying the size of the hyoglossal nerve, which enervates all the intrinsic and most of the extrinsic muscles of the tongue. They estimated the size of the nerve in fossil hominids by determining the cross-sectional area of the hyoglossal canal, the opening in the skull through which the nerve passes. They claim that the hyoglossal canal's area is substantially smaller in living apes than in human beings even when the size of the tongue is factored in, since a larger tongue might imply having a larger nerve. However, their study is flawed because they underestimated the size of the human tongue by a factor of two. When the correct tongue sizes of humans and chimpanzees are compared with hyoglossal canal size there is no difference between the two species (Fitch, personal communication). Since chimpanzees do not talk, relative hyoglossal canal size does not signify the presence or absence of speech. Kay et al. also fail to take into account the body of anatomical evidence demonstrating that the human tongue differs in shape from that of all other mammals and extends well below the oral cavity, as seen in Figure 4–1. The radiographic studies of Russell (1928), Carmody (1937), Chiba and Kajiyama (1941), Perkell (1969), Ladefoged et al. (1972), and Nearey (1979) and MRI studies by Baer et al. (1991) and Story, et al., (1996), among others all show that this is the case. Moreover, the relationship of hyoglossal canal size to speech is moot, DeGusta et al. (1999) show that no correlation exists between the size of the hyoglossal nerve in humans and the number of axons that it contains. DeGusta and his colleagues also show that other nonhuman primates have canals in the modern human range.

6. The length of the oral cavity of the La Chapelle-aux-Saints Neanderthal fossil, which was one factor in Crelin's 1971 reconstruction, can be determined with certainty from either the length of the body of the mandible or the distance between the anterior margin of the foramen magnum, the opening into which the spinal column inserts, and the staphylion, the anterior margin of the skull base. This distance is much greater in the Neanderthal fossil than in any adult human. Exhaustive metrical studies show that the length of this distance in the Neanderthal fossil is completely outside the human range (Howells, 1976, 1989). If you attempt to reconstruct the SVT of this fossil with a pharynx that is equal in length to its oral cavity, the result is an anatomical monster with its larynx positioned in its chest (Lieberman, 1984, 1991). Houghton (1993) proposed

an SVT reconstruction that attempted to solve this problem by fitting a tiny tongue to the La Chapelle-aux-Saints fossil. However, Houghton's proposed Neanderthal tongue would be incapable of propelling food to the back of the Neanderthal mouth, preventing swallowing (Palmer and Hiiemae, 1997; Palmer, 1997). Therefore, Houghton's reconstruction would, if true, account for the extinction of the Neanderthals (Lieberman, 1994c).

7. Fitch (1994, 1997) also shows that human listeners can accurately appraise the size of the person to whom they are listening; the optimal sound is again the vowel [i]. The average fundamental frequency of phonation, F0, which we perceive as the "pitch" of a person's voice, is a surprisingly misleading acoustic cue.
8. Walker and Shipman (1996) note studies of the relative size of the thoracic spinal cord in a *Homo erectus* fossil which indicate that it is smaller than in modern humans. As noted in Chapter 2, the abdominal and chest muscles must execute complex maneuvers to maintain air pressure in a speaker's lungs during the production of speech (Bouhuys, 1974). Moreover, the end of an expiration results in prosodic cues that signal a sentence's end. The duration of expiration during speech production is variable and is usually keyed to sentence length (Lieberman, 1967). The relatively smaller thoracic spinal cord opening, if it is typical of *Homo erectus,* may signify an inability to produce long expirations possessing these prosodic cues, perhaps limiting utterences to short phrases.
9. These "vegetative" deficits are discussed in Lieberman (1975, 1984, 1991).
10. While it is generally the case that humans mate with people speaking the same dialect, it is obvious that this is not always true. Similar events may account for the fact that not all "Neanderthals" appear to resemble completely the "classic" European La Chapelle-aux-Saints fossil. As noted in Lieberman (1984, pp. 315–316), the cranial bases of some fossils classified as Neanderthals have features suggesting that their SVTs may have been more humanlike than the Lieberman and Crelin (1971) reconstruction of the La Chapelle-aux-Saints SVT. The Kebara fossil studied by Arensburg et al. (1990), which was found in Israel, may reflect Neanderthal-AMHS mating. However, since the skull of this fossil is missing, it is difficult to reach a firm conclusion concerning its SVT (Lieberman, 1994b).
11. The lack of correlation between deficits in nonlinguistic gestures and ASL manual gestures noted by Hickok, Bellugi, and Klima (1996) across aphasic sign-language users may reflect different patterns of damage. Brain-imaging techniques currently can show damage to the neuroanatomical structures that support different circuits, but they cannot show whether specific neural circuits are damaged. In some aphasic individuals circuits regulating both modalities may be damaged, in other instances only those regulating ASL. Pooling subjects who show these different patterns can lead to the false conclusion that neuroanatomical structures that regulate motor control have nothing to do with language. The experiment also does not properly control for differences in the level of difficulty in the gestures and signs that were used. Therefore, the conclusion of Hickok, Bellugi, and Klima that their data demonstrate the complete neural independence of language capability from motor control is not warranted.

12. "Sine-wave equivalents" of speech sounds have energy concentrated only at the frequency at which a formant frequency would have occurred in an actual speech signal. As Chapter 1 noted, formant frequencies are usually not directly represented in the acoustic signal; for example, a vowel that has an F0 of 200 Hz will not have any energy at 350 Hz, the first formant frequency of the vowels [i] or [u] for many women, yet listeners will infer the presence of F1 at that frequency. The fact that human listeners will interpret a sine-wave-equivalent signal as speechlike is generally interpreted as signifying the psychological reality of formant frequencies in speech perception.

6. Commentary

1. See Elman et al. (1996) for comprehensive reviews of neural plasticity and the formation of neural circuits during sensitive periods.
2. Categorical perception was discussed in Chapter 1. Detailed discussions can be found in Liberman et al. (1967), Lieberman (1984), and Lieberman and Blumstein (1988).
3. The categorical perception of VOT may be structured by innate constraints, since infants are sensitive to categories that are not present in their native language. However, these innate constraints seem to derive from the properties of the mammalian auditory system (Kuhl, 1981).
4. Liberman's (1979) matrix grammar approximates the power of an augmented transition network (ATN), which has more generative capacity than traditional generative grammars. Associative distributed neural networks have an additional property that is consistent with the recovery of language in aphasic patients suffering damage limited to the cortex (Stuss and Benson, 1986). Associative distributed neural networks are insensitive to local damage; they will continue to function, albeit more slowly and with higher error rates, even after massive damage (Bear et al., 1987).
5. Alexander, Delong, and Crutcher (1992) discuss many studies that predate those noted in Chapters 1 and 4, which support the conclusions reached there concerning the physiology of subcortical-cortical motor control circuits.
6. Studies of specific language impairment (SLI) that focus on syntax often neglect other aspects of language as well as other "nonlinguistic" deficits (e.g., Yamada, 1990). Leonard's (1998) survey of SLI focuses on instances in which linguistic deficits supposedly occur without other cognitive or motor deficits in the absence of brain damage. However, the evidence presented by Leonard is unconvincing; for example, he discusses (pp. 119–132) but then ignores studies that document cognitive and linguistic deficits in children presumed to have SLI. Much of the data that Leonard cites as evidence for SLI derives from studies of children and adults who have difficulty reading or who are slow readers. Moreover, he cites as evidence for SLI studies of reading deficits that do not meet his own criteria for SLI. For example, he discusses (pp. 134–139) the studies of Paula Tallel and her colleagues. However, Tallal (1976) claims that these reading

deficits derive from a general perceptual problem that is not limited to linguistic ability; moreover, reading is a recent invention that cannot be equated with language. The presence of SLI will be uncertain until studies are performed that assess a wide range of behaviors, motor ability, speech, and cognition in children supposed to manifest the condition.

7. Piattelli-Palmarini's declaration of faith, which though it may have been made in jest had an element of truth, was delivered at the 1989 Conference on Genetics and Human Evolution, Florence, Italy.

References

Aiello, L., and R. I. M. Dunbar. 1993. Neocortex size, group size, and the evolution of language. *Current Anthropology* 34: 184–193.

Akshoomoff, N. A., and E. Courchesne. 1992. A new role for the cerebellum in cognitive operations. *Behavioral Neuroscience* 106: 731–738.

Alberch, P. 1989. The logic of monsters. *Geobios* 12: 21–57.

Albert, M. A., R. G. Feldman, and A. L. Willis. 1974. The "subcortical dementia" of progressive supranuclear palsy. *Journal of Neurology, Neurosurgery, and Psychiatry* 37: 121–130.

Aldridge, J. W., K. C. Berridge, M. Herman, and L. Zimmer. 1993. Neuronal coding of serial order: Syntax of grooming in the neostratum. *Psychological Science* 4: 391–393.

Alexander, G. E., M. R. Delong, and M. D. Crutcher. 1992. Do cortical and basal ganglionic motor areas use "motor programs" to control movement? *Behavioral and Brain Sciences* 15: 656–665.

Alexander, G. E., M. R. Delong, and P. L. Strick. 1986. Parallel organization of segregated circuits linking basal ganglia and cortex. *Annual Review of Neuroscience* 9: 357–381.

Alexander, M. P., M. A. Naeser, and C. L. Palumbo. 1987. Correlations of subcortical CT lesion sites and aphasia profiles. *Brain* 110: 961–991.

Anderson, J. A. 1995. *An introduction to neural networks.* Cambridge, Mass.: MIT Press.

Andruski, J., S. E. Blumstein, and M. Burton. 1994. The effect of subphonetic differences on lexical access. *Cognition* 52: 163–187.

Appollonio, I. M., J. Grafman, V. Schwartz, S. Massaquoi, and M. Hallett. 1993. Memory in patients with cerebellar degeneration. *Neurology* 43: 1536–44.

Arensburg, B., L. A. Schepartz, A. M. Tiller, B. Vandermeersch, H. Duday, and Y. Rak. 1990. A reappraisal of the anatomical basis for speech in Middle Palaeolithic hominids. *American Journal of Physical Anthropology* 83: 137–146.

Armstrong, L. E., and I. C. Ward. 1926. *Handbook of English intonation.* Leipzig and Berlin: Teubner.

Artieda, J., M. A. Pastor, F. Lacruz, and J. A. Obeso. 1992. Temporal discrimination is abnormal in Parkinson's disease. *Brain* 115: 199–210.

Atkinson, J. R. 1973. Aspects of intonation in speech: Implications from an experimental study of fundamental frequency. Ph.D. diss., University of Connecticut.

Awh, E., J. Jonides, R. E. Smith, E. H. Schumacher, R. A. Koeppe, and S. Katz. 1996. Dissociation of storage and rehearsal in working memory: Evidence from positron emission tomography. *Psychological Science* 7: 25–31.

Baddeley, A. D. 1986. *Working memory.* Oxford: Clarendon Press.

Baddeley, A. D., and G. Hitch. 1974. Working memory. In *The psychology of learning and motivation,* ed. G. H. Bower. Vol. 8, pp. 47–89. San Diego: Academic Press.

Baddeley, A. D., N. Thomson, and M. Buchanan. 1975. Word length and the structure of short-term memory. *Journal of Verbal Learning and Verbal Behavior* 14: 575–589.

Baer, T., J. C. Gore, L. C. Gracco, and P. W. Nye. 1991. Analysis of vocal tract shape and dimensions using magnetic resonance imaging: Vowels. *Journal of the Acoustical Society of America* 90: 799–828.

Barbujani, G., and R. R. Sokal. 1990. Zones of sharp genetic change in Europe are also linguistic boundaries. *Proceedings of the National Academy of Sciences, USA* 187: 1816–19.

———1991. Genetic population structure of Italy. II: Physical and cultural barriers to gene flow. *American Journal of Human Genetics* 48: 398–411.

Bates, E. 1992. Language development. *Current Opinion in Neurobiology* 2: 180–185.

Bates, E., and J. L. Elman. 1993. Connectionism and the study of change. In *Brain development and cognition: A reader,* ed. M. H. Elman. Oxford: Blackwell.

———1996. Learning rediscovered. *Science* 274: 1849–50.

Bates, E., J. Elman, M. Johnson, A. Karmiloff-Smith, D. Parisi, and K. Plunkett. 1999. On innateness. In *A companion to cognitive science,* ed. W. Bechtael and G. Graham. Oxford: Basil Blackwell.

Bates, E., A. Frederici, and B. Wulfeck. 1987. Comprehension in aphasia: A cross-linguistic study. *Brain and Language* 32: 19–67.

Bates, E., and J. C. Goodman. 1997. On the inseparability of grammar and the lexicon: Evidence from acquisition, aphasia, and real-time processing. *Language and Cognitive Processes* 12: 507–586.

Bates, E., C. Harris, V. Marchman, B. Wulfeck, and M. Kritchevsky. 1995. Production of complex syntax in normal aging and Alzheimer's disease. *Language and Cognitive Processes* 10: 487–539.

Bates, E., and B. MacWhinney. 1989. Functionalism and the competition model. In *The cross-linguistic study of sentence processing,* ed. B. MacWhinney. Cambridge: Cambridge University Press. Pp. 3–37.

Bates, E., D. Thal, and J. Janowsky. 1992. Early language development and its neural correlates. In *Handbook of neuropsychology,* ed. I. Rapin and S. Segalowitz. Vol. 7: *Child neuropsychology.* Amsterdam: Elsevier.

Bates, E., D. Thal, D. Trauner, J. Fenson, D. Aram. J. Eisele, and R. Nass. 1997. From first words to grammar in children with focal brain injury. *Developmental Neuropsychology* 13: 275–343.

Bates, E., S. Vicari, and D. Trauner. 1999. Neural mediation of language development: Perspectives from lesion studies of infants and children. In *Neurodevelopmental disorders: Contributions to a new framework from the cognitive neurosciences,* ed. H. Tager-Flusberg. Cambridge, Mass.: MIT Press. Pp. 533–581.

Bauer, R. H. 1993. Lateralization of neural control for vocalization by the frog (*Rana pipiens*). *Psychobiology* 21: 243–248.

Baum, S. 1988. Syntactic processing in agrammatism: Evidence from lexical decision and grammaticality judgment tasks. *Aphasiology* 2: 117–135.

———1989. On-line sensitivity to local and long-distance syntactic dependencies in Broca's aphasia. *Brain and Language* 37: 327–328.

Baum, S., S. E. Blumstein, M. A. Naeser, and C. L. Palumbo. 1990. Temporal dimensions of consonant and vowel production: An acoustic and CT scan analysis of aphasic speech. *Brain and Language* 37: 327–338.

Baum, S., and W. F. Katz. 1988. Acoustic analysis of compensatory articulation in children. *Journal of the Acoustical Society of America* 84: 1662–68.

Bavelier, D., D. Corina, V. P. Clark, P. Jezzard, A. Prinster, A. Karni, A. Lalwani, J. Rauschecker, R. Turner, and H. Neville. 1995. Sentence reading: an fMRI study at 4T. *Human Brain Mapping* 1 (suppl.): 239.

Bayles, K., and C. K. Tomoeda. 1983. Confrontation namimg in dementia. *Brain and Language* 19: 98–114.

Bear, M. F., B. W. Conners, and M. A. Paradiso. 1996. *Neuroscience: Exploring the brain.* Baltimore: Williams and Wilkins.

Bear, M. F., L. N. Cooper, and F. F. Ebner. 1987. A physiological basis for a theory of synaptic modification. *Science* 237: 42–48.

Beatty, W. W., R. D. Staton, W. S. Weir, N. Monson, and H. A. Whittaker. 1989. Cognitive disturbances in Parkinson's disease. *Journal of Geriatric Psychiatry and Neurology* 2: 22–33.

Beckman, M. E., T.-P. Jung, S.-H. Lee, K. de Jong, A. K. Krishnamurthy, S. C. Ahalt, K. B. Cohen, and M. J. Collins. 1995. Variability in the production of quantal vowels revisited. *Journal of the Acoustical Society of America* 97: 471–489.

Bell, A. G. 1867. *Visible speech.* London: Simpkin and Marshall.

Bell, C. G., H. Fujisaki, J. M. Heinz, K. N. Stevens, and A. S. House. 1961. Reduction of speech spectra by analysis-by-synthesis techniques. *Journal of the Acoustical Society of America* 33: 1725–36.

Bellugi, U., H. Poizner, and E. S. Klima. 1983. Brain organization for language: Clues from sign aphasia. *Human Neurobiology* 2: 155–170.

Berridge, K. C., and I. Q. Whitshaw. 1992. Cortex, striatum, and cerebellum: Control of serial order in a grooming sequence. *Experimental Brain Research* 90: 275–290.

Bickerton, D. 1990. *Language and species.* Chicago: University of Chicago Press.

———1998a. Review of *Eve spoke: Human language and human evolution. New York Times Book Review,* March 3.

———1998b. From protolanguage to language. Paper presented at the Second International Conference on the Evolution of Language, London, April.

Blackwell, A., and E. Bates. 1995. Inducing agrammatic profiles in normals: Evidence for the selective vunerability of morphology under cognitive resource limitation. *Journal of Cognitive Neuroscience* 7: 28–257.

Bloomfield, L. 1933. *Language*. New York: Holt.

Blumstein, S. E. 1994. The neurobiology of the sound structure of language. In *The cognitive neurosciences,* ed. M. S. Gazzaniga. Cambridge, Mass.: MIT Press.

———1995. The neurobiology of language. In *Speech, language and communication,* ed. J. Miller and P. D. Elmas. San Diego: Academic Press. Pp. 339–370.

Blumstein, S. E., W. Cooper, H. Goodglass, H. Statlender, and J. Gottleib. 1980. Production deficits in aphasia: A voice-onset time analysis. *Brain and Language* 9: 153–170.

Blumstein, S. E., and K. N. Stevens. 1979. Acoustic invariance in speech production: Evidence from measurements of the spectral properties of stop consonants. *Journal of the Acoustical Society of America* 66: 1001–17.

———1980. Perceptual invariance and onset spectra for stop consonants in different vowel environments. *Journal of the Acoustical Society of America* 67: 648–662.

Boesch, C., and H. Boesch. 1993. Aspects of transmission of tool-use in wild chimpanzees. In *Tools, language and cognition in human evolution,* ed. K. R. Gibson and T. Ingold. Cambridge: Cambridge University Press. Pp. 171–184.

Bouhuys, A. 1974. *Breathing*. New York: Grune and Stratton.

Bradshaw, J. L., and N. C. Nettleton. 1981. The nature of hemispheric lateralization in man. *Behavioral and Brain Sciences* 4: 51–92.

Broca, P. 1861. Remarques sur le siège de la faculté de la parole articulée, suivies d'une observation d'aphémie (perte de parole). *Bulletin de la Société d'Anatomie* (Paris) 6: 330–357.

Brodmann, K. 1908. Beitrage zur histologischen Lokalisation der Grosshirnrinde. VII. Mitteilung: Die cytoarchitektonische Cortexgleiderung der Halbaffen (Lemuriden). *Journal für Psychologie und Neurologie* 10: 287–334.

———1909. *Vergleichende Histolgisiche Lokalisation der Groshirnrinde in iheren Prinzipen Dargestellt auf Grund des Zellenbaues.* Leipzig: Barth.

———1912. Ergebnisse uber die vergleichende histologische Lokalisation der Grosshirnrinde mit besonderer Berucksichtigung des Stirnhirns. *Anatomischer Anzeiger* 41 (suppl.): 157–216.

Brozoski, T. J., R. M. Brown, H. E. Rosvold, and P. S. Goldman-Rakic. 1979. Cognitive deficit caused by regional depletion of dopamins in prefrontal cortex of rhesus monkey. *Science* 205: 929–931.

Bruyn, G. W. 1969. Huntington's chorea: Historical, clinical, and laboratory synopsis. In *Handbook of clinical neurology,* ed. P. J. Linken and G. W. Bruyn. Vol. 13, pp. 298–378. Amsterdam: North Holland.

Bunge, M. 1984. Philosophical problems in linguistics. *Erkenntnis* 21: 107–173.

———1985. From mindless neuroscience and brainless psychology to neuropsychology. *Annals of Theoretical Psychology* 3: 115–133.

Burling, R. 1993. Primate calls, human language, and nonverbal communication. *Current Anthropology* 34: 1–37.

Calvin, W. H. 1993. The unitary hypothesis: A common neural circuitry for novel manipulations, language, plan-ahead, and throwing? In *Tools, language, and cognition in human evolution*, ed. K. R. Gibson and T. Ingold. Cambridge: Cambridge University Press. Pp. 230–250.

Calvin, W. H., and D. Bickerton. 2000. *Lingua ex machina: Reconciling Darwin and Chomsky with the human brain.* Cambridge, Mass.: MIT Press.

Caplan, D. 1987. *Neurolinguistics and linguistic aphasiology: An introduction.* Cambridge: Cambridge University Press.

Caplan, D., and N. Hildebrandt. 1988. *Disorders of syntactic comprehension.* Cambridge, Mass.: MIT Press.

Caplan, D., and G. S. Waters. 1990. Short-term memory and language comprehension: A critcal review of the neuropsychological literature. In *Neuropsychological impairments of S.T.M.*, ed. G. Villar and T. Shallice. London: Cambridge University Press.

Capranica, R. R. 1965. *The evoked vocal response of the bullfrog.* Cambridge, Mass.: MIT Press.

Carew, T. J., E. T. Waters, and E. R. Kandel. 1981. Associative learning in *Aplysia:* Cellular correlates supporting a conditioned fear hypothesis. *Science* 211: 501–503.

Carmody, F. 1937. X-ray studies of speech articulation. *University of California Publications in Modern Philology* 20: 187–237.

Carramaza, A., and A. E. Hillis. 1990. Lexical organization of nouns and verbs in the brain. *Nature* 349: 788–790.

Carré, R., B. Lindblom, and P. MacNeilage. 1994. Acoustic factors in the evolution of the human vocal tract. *Journal of the Acoustical Society of America* 95: 2924.

Cheney, D. L., and R. M. Seyfarth. 1990. *How monkeys see the world: Inside the mind of aother species.* Chicago: University of Chicago Press.

Chiba, T., and J. Kajiyama. 1941. *The vowel: Its nature and structure.* Tokyo: Tokyo-Kaisekan.

Chomsky, N. 1957. *Syntactic structures.* The Hague: Mouton.

———1966. *Cartesian Linguistics.* New York: Harper and Row.

———1972. *Language and mind.* Enl. ed. New York: Harcourt, Brace and World.

———1976. On the nature of language. In *Origins and evolution of language and speech*, ed. H. B. Steklis, S. R. Harnad, and J. Lancaster. New York: New York Academy of Sciences. Pp. 46–57.

———1980a. Initial states and steady states. In *Language and learning: The debate between Jean Piaget and Noam Chomsky*, ed. M. Piattelli-Palmarini. Cambridge, Mass.: Harvard University Press. Pp. 107–130.

———1980b. Rules and representations. *Behavioral and Brain Sciences* 3: 1–61.

———1981. *Lectures on government and binding.* Dordrecht: Foris.

———1986. *Knowledge of language: Its nature, origin, and use.* New York: Praeger.

———1995. *The minimalist program.* Cambridge, Mass.: MIT Press.

Chomsky, N., and M. Halle. 1968. *The sound pattern of English.* New York: Harper and Row.

Churchland, P. M. 1995. *The engine of reason, the seat of the soul: A philosophical journey into the brain.* Cambridge, Mass.: MIT Press.

Classen, J., J. Liepert, S. P. Wise, M. Hallet, and L. G. Cohen. 1998. Rapid plasticity of human cortical movement representation induced by practice. *Journal of Neurophysiology* 79: 1117–23.

Cohen, H., S. Bouchard, P. Scherzer, and H. Whittaker. 1994. Language and verbal reasoning in Parkinson's disease. *Neuropsychiatry, Neuropsychology, and Behavioral Neurology* 7: 166–175.

Cohen, L. G., P. Celnik, A. Pascual-Leone, B. Corwell, L. Faiz, J. Dambrosia, M. Honda, N. Sadato, C. Gerloff, M. D. Catata, and M. Hallet. 1997. Functional relevance of cross-modal plasticity in blind humans. *Nature* 389: 180–184.

Courtney, S. M., L. Petit, M. M. Jose, L. G. Ungerleider, and J. V. Haxby. 1998. An area specialized for spatial working memory in human frontal cortex. *Science* 279: 1347–51.

Croft, W. 1991. *Syntactic categories and grammatical relations.* Chicago: University of Chicago Press.

Crosson, B. 1984. Role of the dominant thalamus in language: A review. *Psychological Bulletin* 90: 491–517.

Crutcher, M. D., and G. E. Alexander. 1990. Movement-related neuronal activity coding either direction or muscle pattern in three motor areas of the monkey. *Journal of Neurophysiology* 64: 151–163.

Crutcher, M. D., and M. R. Delong. 1984. Single-cell studies of the primate putamen: Relations to direction of movement and pattern of muscular activity. *Experimental Brain Research* 53: 244–258.

Cummings, J. L. 1993. Frontal-subcortical circuts and human behavior. *Archives of Neurology* 50: 873–880.

Cummings, J. L., and D. F. Benson. 1984. Subcortical dementia: Review of an emerging concept. *Archives of Neurology* 41: 874–879.

Cunnington, R., R. Iansek, J. L. Bradshaw, and J. G. Phillips. 1995. Movement-related potentials in Parkinson's disease: Presence and predictability of temporal and spatial cues. *Brain* 118: 935–950.

Curtiss, S. 1977. *Genie: A psycholinguistic study of a modern-day "wild child."* New York: Academic Press.

Cymerman, A., P. Lieberman, J. Hochstadt, P. B. Rock, G. E. Butterfield, and L. G. Moore. 1999. Speech motor control and the development of acute mountain sickness. U.S. Army Research Institute of Environmental Medicine, Technical Report no. T99-5, AD A360764. Alexandria, Va.: Defense Technical Information Center.

Dale, P. S., E. Simonoff, D. V. M. Bishop, T. C. Eley, B. Oliver, T. S. Price, S. Purcell, J. Stevenson, and R. Plomin. 1998. Genetic influence on language delay in 2-year-olds. *Nature Neuroscience* 1: 324–328.

Damasio, A. R., and D. Tranel. 1993. Nouns and verbs are retrieved with differently distributed neural systems. *Proceedings of the National Academy of Sciences, USA* 90: 4957–60.

Damasio, H. 1991. Neuroanatomical correlates of the aphasias. In *Acquired aphasia,* ed. M. T. Sarno. 2d ed. New York: Academic Press.

Damasio, H., T. J. Grabowski, D. Tranel, R. D. Hichwa, and A. R. Damasio. 1996. A neural basis for lexical retrieval. *Nature* 380: 409–505.

Daneman, M., and P. A. Carpenter. 1980. Individual differences in comprehension and producing words in context. *Journal of Verbal Learning and Behavior* 19: 450–466.

D'Antonia, R., J. C. Baron, Y. Samson, M. Serdaru, F. Viader, Y. Agid, and J. Cambier. 1985. Subcortical dementia: Frontal cortex hypometabolism detected by positron tomography in patients with progressive supranuclear palsy. *Brain* 108: 785–799.

Darwin, C. 1859. *On the origin of species.* Facsimile ed. Cambridge, Mass.: Harvard University Press, 1964.

Davidson, I., and W. Noble. 1993. Tools and language in human evolution. In *Tools, language, and cognition in human evolution,* ed. K. R. Gibson and T. Ingold. Cambridge: Cambridge University Press. Pp. 363–388.

Deacon, T. W. 1988. Human brain evolution. II: Embryology and brain allometry. In *Intelligence and evolutionary biology,* ed. H. J. Jerison and I. Jerison. NATO ASI Series. Berlin: Springer. Pp. 383–416.

———1997. *The symbolic species: The co-evolution of language and the brain.* New York: W. W. Norton.

DeGusta, D., W. H. Gilbert, and S. P. Turner. 1999. Hypoglossal canal size and hominid speech. *Proceedings of the National Academy of Sciences* 96: 1800–04.

DeLong, M. R. 1993. Overview of basal ganglia function. In *Role of the cerebellum and basal ganglia in voluntary movement,* ed. N. Mano, I. Hamada, and M. R. DeLong. Amsterdam: Elsevier.

Denneberg, V. H. 1981. Hemispheric laterality in animals and the effects of early experience. *Behavioral and Brain Sciences* 4: 1–50.

D'Errico, F., J. Zilhao, M. Julien, D. Baffier, J. and Pelegrin. 1998. Neanderthal acculturation in western Europe? A critical review of the evidence and its interpretation. *Current Anthropology* 39 (suppl.): 1–44.

D'Esposito, M., and M. P. Alexander. 1995. Subcortical aphasia: Distinct profiles following left putaminal hemorrhage. *Neurology* 45: 38–41.

D'Esposito, M., J. A. Detre, D. C. Alsop, R. K. Shin, S. Atlas, and M. Grossman. 1995. The neural basis of the central executive system of working memory. *Science* 378: 279–281.

Donald, M. 1991. *Origins of the modern mind.* Cambridge, Mass.: Harvard University Press.

Donoghue, J. P. 1995. Plasticity of adult sensorimotor representations. *Current Opinion in Neurobiology* 5: 749–754.

Driver, J. 1996. Enhancement of selective listening by illusory mislocation of speech sounds due to lip-reading. *Nature* 381: 66–68.

Dronkers, N. F., J. K. Shapiro, B. Redfern, and R. T. Knight. 1992. The role of Broca's area in Broca's aphasia. *Journal of Clinical and Experimental Neuropsychology* 14: 198.

Edelman, G. M. 1987. *Neural Darwinism.* New York: Basic Books.

Eimas, P. D. 1974. Auditory and linguistic processing of cues for place of articulation by infants. *Perception and Psychophysics* 16: 513–521.

Elbert, T., C. Pantev, C. Wienbruch, B. Rockstroh, and E. Taub. 1995. Increased cortical representation of the fingers of the left hand in string players. *Science* 270: 305–307.

Elman, J. 1996. Associative learning in recurrent neural nets. Lecture, Brown University, April 23.

———In press. Distributed representations, simple recurrent networks, and grammatical structure. *Machine Learning.*

Elman, J., E. Bates, M. Johnson, A. Karmiloff-Smith, D. Parisi, and K. Plunkett. 1996. *Rethinking innateness: A connectionist perspective on development.* Cambridge, Mass.: MIT Press.

Engen, E., and T. Engen. 1983. *Rhode Island Test of Language Structure.* Baltimore: University Park Press.

Evarts, E. V. 1973. Motor cortex reflexes associated with learned movement. *Science* 179: 501–503.

Falk, D. 1975. Comparative anatomy of the larynx in man and the chimpanzee: Implications for language in Neanderthal. *American Journal of Physical Anthropology* 43: 123–132.

Fant, G. 1960. *Acoustic theory of speech production.* The Hague: Mouton.

Fernald, A., T. Taeschner, J. Dunn, M. Papousek, B. de Boysson-Bardies, and I. Fukui. 1989. A cross-language study of prosodic modifications in mothers' and fathers' speech to preverbal infants. *Journal of Child Language* 16: 477–501.

Ferreira, F., and C. Clifton. 1986. The independence of syntactic processing. *Journal of Memory and Language* 25: 1–18.

Fiez, J. A., F. E. Peterson, M. K. Cheney, and M. E. Raichle. 1992. Impaired non-motor learning and error detection associated with cerebellar damage: A single case study. *Brain* 115: 155–178.

Fillmore, C. J., P. Kay, and C. O'Conner. 1988. Regularity and idiomaticity in grammatical constructions: The case of LET Alone. *Language* 64: 501–538.

Fink, G. R., R. S. Frackowiak, U. Pietrzyk, and R. E. Passingham. 1997. Multiple nonprimary motor areas in the human cortex. *Journal of Neurophysiology* 77: 2164–74.

Fisher, S. E., F. Vargha-Khadem, K. E. Watkins, A. P. Monaco, and M. E. Pembrey. 1998. Localization of a gene implicated in a severe speech and language disorder. *Nature Genetics* 18: 168–170.

Fitch, W. T., III. 1994. Vocal tract length and the evolution of language. Ph.D. diss., Brown University.

———1997. Vocal tract length and formant frequency dispersion correlate with body size in macaque monkeys. *Journal of the Acoustical Society of America* 102: 1213–22.

Flowers, K. A., and C. Robertson. 1985. The effects of Parkinson's disease on the ability to maintain a mental set. *Journal of Neurology, Neurosurgery, and Psychiatry* 48: 517–529.

Fodor, J. 1983. *Modularity of mind.* Cambridge, Mass.: MIT Press.

Frayer, D. W., M. H. Wolpoff, A. G. Thorne, F. H. Smith, and G. G. Pope. 1993. Theories of modern human origins: The paleontological test. *American Anthropologist* 95: 14–50.

Frishkopf, L. S., and M. H. Goldstein Jr. 1963. Responses to acoustic stimuli from single units in the eighth nerve of the bullfrog. *Journal of the Acoustical Society of America* 35: 1219–28.

Fujimura, O., and Y. Kakita. 1979. Remarks on quantitative description of lingual articulation. In *Frontiers of speech communication research,* ed. B. Lindblom and S. Ohman. London: Academic Press. Pp. 17–24.

Funahashi, S., C. J. Brule, and P. S. Goldman-Rakic. 1993. Dorsolateral prefrontal lesions and oculomotor delayed response performance: Evidence for mnemonic "scotomas." *Journal of Neuroscience* 13: 1479–97.

Fuster, J. M. 1989. *The prefrontal cortex: Anatomy, physiology, and neuropsychology of the frontal lobe.* 2d ed. New York: Raven Press.

Galaburda, A., G. Sherman, G. Rosen, F. Abolitz, and N. Geschwind. 1985. Developmental dyslexia: Four consecutive patients with cortical anomolies. *Annals of Neurology* 18: 222–233.

Gall, F. J. 1809. *Recherches sur le système nerveux.* Paris: J. B. Balliere.

Gannon, P. J., R. L. Holloway, D. C. Broadfield, and A. R. Braun. 1998. Asymmetry of Chimpanzee plenum temporale: Humanlike pattern of Wernicke's brain language area homolog. *Science* 279: 220–222.

Gardner, R. A., and B. T. Gardner. 1969. Teaching sign language to a chimpanzee. *Science* 165: 664–672.

———1984. A vocabulary test for chimpanzees (*Pan troglodytes*). *Journal of Comparative Psychology* 4: 381–404.

———1994. Development of phrases in the utterances of children and cross-fostered chimpanzees. In *The etholoical roots of culture,* ed. R. A. Gardner, B. T. Gardner, B. Chiarelli, and R. Plooj. Dordrecht: Kluwer Academic Publishers. Pp. 223–255.

Gardner, R. A., B. T. Gardner, and T. E. Van Cantfort. 1989. *Teaching sign language to chimpanzees.* Albany: State University of New York Press.

Gathercole, S. E., and A. D. Baddeley. 1993. *Working memory and language.* Hillside, Pa.: Lawrence Erlbaum Associates.

Geschwind, N. 1970. The organization of language and the brain. *Science* 170: 940–944.

Geschwind, N., and W. Levitsky. 1968. Human brain: Asymmetries in the temporal speech area. *Science* 161: 186–187.

Goel, V., and J. Grafman. 1995. Are frontal lobes implicated in "planning" functions: Interpreting data from the Tower of Hanoi. *Neuropsychologia* 33: 623–642.

Goldberg, A. E. 1995. *Constructions: A construction grammar approach to argument structure.* Chicago: University of Chicago Press.

Goldin-Meadow, S. 1993. When does gesture become language? A study of gesture used as the primary communication by deaf children of hearing parents. In *Tools, language, and cognition in human evolution,* ed. K. R. Gibson and T. Ingold. Cambridge: Cambridge University Press. Pp. 63–85.

Goldin-Meadow, S., and C. Mylander. 1998. Spontaneous sign systems created by deaf children in two cultures. *Nature* 391: 279–281.

Goldman-Rakic, P. S. 1987. Circuitry of primate prefrontal cortex and the regulation of behavior by representational memory. In *Handbook of physiology.* Vol. 5: *The nervous system,* ed. F. Plum and V. Mountcastle. Bethesda, Md.: American Physiological Society. Pp. 373–417.

Goldstein, K. 1948. *Language and language disturbances.* New York: Grune and Stratton.

Goodall, J. 1986. *The chimpanzees of Gombe: Patterns of behavior.* Cambridge, Mass.: Harvard University Press.

Goodglass, H., and E. Kaplan. 1983. *Boston Diagnostic Aphasia Examination (BDAE).* Malvern, Pa.: Lea and Febiger.

Gopnik, A., and A. N. Meltzoff. 1986. Words, plans, things, and locations: Interactions between semantic and cognitive development in the one-word stage. In *The development of word meaning,* ed. S. A. Kuczaj and M. D. Barrett. New York: Springer Verlag.

Gopnick, M. 1990. Dysphasia in an extended family. *Nature* 344: 715.

Gopnick, M., and M. Crago. 1991. Familial segregation of a developmental language disorder. *Cognition* 39: 1–50.

Gordon, W. P., and J. Illes. 1987. Neurolinguistic characteristics of language production in Huntington's disease: A preliminary report. *Brain and Language* 31: 1–10.

Gotham, A. M., R. G. Brown, and C. D. Marsden. 1988. "Frontal" cognitive function in patients with Parkinson's disease "on" and "off" Levadopa. *Brain* 111: 199–321.

Gottlieb, G. 1975. Development of species identification in ducklings. I: Nature of perceptual deficits caused by embryonic auditory deprivation. *Journal of Comparative and Physiological Psychology* 89: 387–389.

Gould, S. J. 1977. *Ontogeny and phylogeny.* Cambridge, Mass.: Harvard University Press.

Gould, S. J., and N. Eldridge. 1977. Punctuated equilibria: The tempo and mode of evolution reconsidered. *Paleobiology* 3: 115–151.

Graco, V., and J. Abbs. 1985. Dynamic control of the perioral system during speech: Kinematic analyses of autogenic and nonautogenic sensorimotor processes. *Journal of Neurophysiology* 54: 418–432.

Grafman, J. 1989. Plans, actions, and mental sets: The role of the frontal lobes. In *Integrating theory and practice in clinical neuropsychology,* ed. E. Perecman. Hilldise, N.J.: Lawrence Erlbaum Associates.

Grafman, J., I. Litvan, S. Massaquoi, M. Stewart, A. Sirigu, and M. Hallet. 1992. Cognitive planning deficit in patients with cerebellar atrophy. *Neurology* 42: 1493–1506.

Graybiel, A. M., T. Aosaki, A. W. Flaherty, and M. Kimura. 1994. The basal ganglia and adaptive motor control. *Science* 265: 1826–31.

Graziano, M. S. A., G. S. Yap, and C. G. Gross. 1994. Coding of visual space by premotor neurons. *Science* 266: 1054–57.

Greenberg, J. 1963. *Universals of language.* Cambridge, Mass.: MIT Press.

Greenfield, P. M. 1991. Language, tools, and brain: The ontogeny and phylogeny of hierarchically organized sequential behavior. *Behavioral and Brain Sciences* 14: 531–577.

Greenwalt, C. A. 1968. *Bird song: Acoustics and physiology.* Washington, D.C.: Smithsonian Institution Press.

Grieser, D. L., and P. K. Kuhl. 1988. Maternal speech to infants in a tonal language: Support for universal prosodic features in motherese. *Developmental Psychology* 24: 14–20.

———1989. Categorization of speech by infants: Support for speech-sound prototypes. *Developmental Psychology* 25: 577–588.

Grosmangin, C. 1979. *Base du crane et pharynx dans leur rapports avec l'appareil de langage articulé.* Mémoires du Laboratoire d'Anatomie de la Faculté de Medicine de Paris, no. 40-1979.

Gross, C. 1995. The representation of space in the brain. Lecture, Brown University, January 26.

Grossman, M., S. Carvell, S. Gollomp, M. B. Stern, G. Vernon, and H. I. Hurtig. 1991. Sentence comprehension and praxis deficits in Parkinson's disease. *Neurology* 41: 160–1628.

Grossman, M., S. Carvell, S. Gollomp, M. B. Stern, Reivich, D. Morrison, A. Alavi, and H. L. Hurtig. 1993. Cognitive and physiological substrates of impaired sentence processing in Parkinson's disease. *Journal of Cognitive Neuroscience* 5: 480–498.

Hales, R. E., and S. C. Yudofsky. 1987. *Textbook of neuropsychiatry.* Washington, D.C.: American Psychiatric Press.

Harrington, D. L., and K. Y. Haaland. 1991. Sequencing in Parkinson's disease: Abnormalities in programming and controlling movement. *Brain* 114: 99–115.

Hata, Y., and M. P. Stryker. 1994. Control of thalamocortical afferent rearrangement by postsynaptic activity in developing visual cortex. *Science* 263: 1732–35.

Hauser, M. D. 1996. *The evolution of communication.* Cambridge, Mass.: MIT Press.

Hayes, K. J., and C. Hayes. 1951. The intellectual development of a home-raised chimpanzee. *Proceedings of the American Philosophical Society* 95: 105–109.

Hebb, D. O. 1949. *The organization of behavior: A neuropsychological theory.* New York: Wiley.

Hellwag, C. 1781. *De formatione loquelae.* Diss., Tübingen.

Herrnstein, R. J. 1979. Acquisition, generalization, and discrimination of a natural concept. *Journal of Experimental Psychology and Animal Behavioral Processes* 5: 116–129.

Herrnstein, R. J., and P. A. de Villiers. 1980. Fish as a natural category for people and pigeons. In *The psychology of learning and motivation,* ed. G. H. Bower. Vol. 14, pp. 59–95. New York: Academic Press.

Herrnstein, R. J., and C. Murray. 1994. *The bell curve: Intelligence and class structure in American life.* New York: Free Press.

Hewes, G. W. 1973. Primate communication and the gestural origin of language. *Current Anthropology* 14: 5–24.

Hickok, G., U. Bellugi, and E. S. Klima. 1996. The neurobiology of sign language and its implications for the neural basis of language. *Nature* 381: 699–720.

Hirsch, I., and C. E. Sherrick. 1961. Perceived order in different sense modalities. *Journal of Experimental Psychology* 62: 423–432.

Hitch, G. J., and A. D. Baddeley. 1976. Verbal reasoning and working memory. *Quarterly Journal of Experimental Psychology* 28: 603–621.

Hoehn, M. M., and M. D. Yahr. 1967. Parkinsonism: Onset, progression, and mortality. *Neurology* 17: 427–442.

Holloway, R. L. 1995. Evidence for POT expansion in early *Homo:* A pretty theory with ugly (or no) paleoneurological facts. *Behavioral and Brain Sciences* 18: 191–193.

Hoover, J. E., and P. L. Strick. 1993. Multiple output channels in the basal ganglia. *Science* 259: 819–821.

Houghton, P. 1993. Neanderthal supralaryngeal vocal tract. *American Journal of Physical Anthropology* 90: 139–146.

Howells, W. W. 1976. Neanderthal man: Facts and figures. In *Proceedings of the Ninth International Congress of Anthropological and Ethnological Sciences, Chicago 1973.* The Hague: Mouton.

———1989. *Skull shapes and the map: Craniometric analyses in the dispersion of modern Homo.* Papers of the Peabody Museum of Archaeology and Ethnology, Harvard University, vol. 79.

Hublin, J.-J., F. Spoor, M. Braun, F. Zonneveld, and S. Condemi. 1996. A late Neanderthal associated with Upper Paleolithic artifacts. *Nature* 381: 224–226.

Hulme, C., N. Thomson, C. Muir, and A. Lawrence. 1984. Speech rate and the development of short-term memory span. *Journal of Experimental Child Psychology* 47: 241–253.

Illes, J., E. J. Metter, W. R. Hanson, and S. Iritani. 1988. Language production in Parkinson's disease: Acoustic and linguistic considerations. *Brain and Language* 33: 146–160.

Ivry, R. B., and S. W. Keele. 1989. Timing functions of the cerebellum. *Journal of Cognitive Neuroscience* 1: 134–150.

Jackendoff, R. 1994. *Patterns in the mind: Language and human nature.* New York: Basic Books.

Jakobson, R. 1940. Kindersprache, Aphasie und allgemeine Lautgesetze. In *Selected writings.* The Hague: Mouton. Translated by A. R. Keiler in *Child language, aphasia, and phonological universals.* The Hague: Mouton, 1968.

Jakobson, R., C. G. M. Fant, and M. Halle. 1952. *Preliminaries to speech analysis.* Cambridge, Mass.: MIT Press.

Jellinger, K. 1990. New developments in the pathology of Parkinson's disease. In *Advances in neurology.* Vol. 53: *Parkinson's disease: Anatomy, pathology, and therapy,* ed. M. B. Streifler, A. D. Korezyn, J. Melamed, and M. B. H. Youdim. New York: Raven Press. Pp. 1–15.

Jerison, H. J. 1973. *Evolution of the brain and intelligence.* New York: Academic Press.

Johnson, J. S., and E. L. Newport. 1989. Critical period effects in second language learning: The influence of maturational state on the acquisition of English as a second language. *Cognitive Psychology* 21: 60–99.

Jones, D. 1932. *An outline of English phonetics.* 3d ed. New York: Dutton.

Just, M. A., and P. A. Carpenter. 1992. A capacity theory of comprehension: Individual differences in working memory. *Psychological Review* 99: 122–149.

Just, M. A., P. A. Carpenter, T. A. Keller, W. F. M. Eddy, and K. R. Thulborn. 1996. Brain activation modulated by sentence comprehension. *Science* 274: 114–116.

Kagan, J. 1989. *Unstable ideas: Temperament, cognition, and self.* Cambridge, Mass.: Harvard University Press.

Kagan, J., J. S. Reznick, and N. Snidman. 1988. Biological bases of childhood shyness. *Science* 240: 167–171.

Karni, A., G. Meyer, P. Jezzard, M. M. Adams, R. Turner, and L. G. Ungerleider. 1995. Functional MRI evidence for adult motor cortex plasticity during motor skill learning. *Nature* 377: 155–158.

Karni, A., G. Meyer, C. Rey-Hipolito, P. Jezzard, M. M. Adams and L. G. Ungerleider. 1998. The acquisition of skilled motor performance: Fast and slow experience-driven changes in primary motor cortex. *Proceedings of the National Academy of Sciences, USA* 953: 861–868.

Katz, W. F. 1988. Anticipatory coarticulation in aphasia: Acoustic and perceptual data. *Brain and Language* 35: 340–368.

Katz, W., J. Machetanz, U. Orth, and P. Schonle. 1990a. A kinematic analysis of anticipatory coarticulation in the speech of anterior aphasic subjects using electromagnetic articulography. *Brain and Language* 38: 555–575.

———1990b. Anticipatory labial coarticulation in the speech of German-speaking anterior aphasic subjects: Acoustic analyses. *Journal of Neurolinguistics* 5: 295–320.

Kay, R. F., M. Cartmill, and M. Balow. 1998. The hypoglossal canal and the origin of human vocal behavior. *Proceedings of the National Academy of Sciences, USA* 95: 5417–19.

Kelso, J. A. S., A. Fuchs, R. Lancaster, T. Holroyd, D. Cheyne, and H. Weinberg. 1998. Dynamic cortical activity in the human brain reveals motor equivalence. *Nature* 392: 814–818.

Kemper, S. 1992. Language and aging. In *The handbook of aging and cognition,* ed. F. I. M. Craik and T. A. Salthouse. Hillsdale, N.J.: Lawrence Erlbaum Associates. Pp. 213–272.

Kempler, D. 1988. Lexical and pantomime abilities in Alzheimer's disease. *Aphasiology* 2: 147–159.

Kempler, D., S. Curtiss, and C. Jackson. 1987. Syntactic preservation in Alzheimer's disease. *Journal of Speech and Hearing Research* 30: 343–350.

Kent, R., and J. Rosenbek. 1983. Acoustic patterns of apraxia of speech. *Journal of Speech and Hearing Research* 26: 231–248.

Kermadi, I., and J. P. Joseph. 1995. Activity in the caudate nucleus of monkey during spatial sequencing. *Journal of Neurophysiology* 74: 911–933.

Kim, S. G, K. Ugurbil, and P. L. Strick. 1994. Activation of a cerebellar output nucleus during cognitive procesing. *Science* 265: 949–951.

Kimura, D. 1979. Neuromotor mechanisms in the evolution of human communication. In *Neurobiology of social communication in primates,* ed. H. D. Steklis and M. J. Raleigh. New York: Academic Press.

———1993. *Neuromotor mechanisms in human communication.* Oxford: Oxford University Press.

Kimura, M., T. Aosaki, and A. Graybiel. 1993. Role of basal ganglia in the acquisition and initiation of learned movement. In *Role of the cerebellum and basal ganglia in voluntary movements,* ed. N. Mano, I. Hamada, and M. R. DeLong. Amsterdam: Elsevier. Pp. 71–75.

King, J., and M. A. Just. 1991. Individual differences in syntactic comprehension: The role of working memory. *Journal of Memory and Learning* 30: 580–602.

Kingdon, J. 1993. *Self-made man.* New York: John Wiley.

Klatt, D. H., and R. A. Stefanski. 1974. How does a mynah bird imitate human speech? *Journal of the Acoustical Society of America* 55: 822–832.

Klein, D., B. Milner, R. J. Zatorre, E. Meyer, and A. C. Evans. 1995. The neural substrates underlying word generation: A bilingual functional imaging study. *Proceedings of the National Academy of Sciences, USA* 92: 2899–2903.

Klein, D., R. J. Zatorre, B. Milner, E. Meyer, and A. C. Evans. 1994. Left putaminal activation when speaking a second language: Evidence from PET. *NeuroReport* 5: 2295–97.

Kohonen, T. 1984. *Self-organization and associative memory.* New York: Springer Verlag.

Kosslyn, S. M., A. Pascual-Leone, O. Felician, S. Camposano, J. P. Keenan, W. L. Thompson, G. Ganis, K. E. Sukel, and N. M. Alpert. 1999. The role of area 17 in visual imagery: Convergent evidence from PET and rTMS. *Science* 284: 167–170.

Krakauer, J. 1997. *Into thin air.* New York: Villard.

Kramer, S. S. 1991. Swallowing in children. In *Normal and abnormal swallowing: Imaging in diagnosis and therapy,* ed. B. Jones and M. W. Donner. New York: Springer Verlag. Pp. 173–188.

Krams, M., M. F. Rushworth, M. P. Deiber, R. S. Frackowiak, and R. E. Passingham. 1998. The preparation, execution, and suppression of copied movements in the human brain. *Experimental Brain Research* 120: 386–398.

Kraus, N., T. J. McGee, T. D. Carrell, S. G. Zecker, T. G. Nicol, and D. B. Koch. 1996. Auditory neurophysiologic responses and discrimination deficits in children with learning problems. *Science* 273: 971–973.

Krings, M., A. Stone, R. W. Schmitz, H. Krainitzki, M. Stoneking, and S. Paabo. 1997. Neanderthal DNA sequences and the origin of modern humans. *Cell* 90: 19–30.

Kuhl, P. K. 1981. Discrimination of speech by nonhuman animals: Basic auditory sensitivities conducive to the perception of speech-sound categories. *Journal of the Acoustical Society of America* 70: 340–349.

Kuhl, P. K., K. A. Williams, F. Lacerda, K. N. Stevens, and B. Lindblom. 1992. Linguistic experience alters phonetic perception in infants by 6 months of age. *Science* 255: 606–608.

Kutas, M. 1997. Views on how the electrical activity that the brain generates reflects the functions of different language structures. *Psychophysiology* 34: 383–398.

Ladefoged, P., and D. E. Broadbent. 1957. Information conveyed by vowels. *Journal of the Acoustical Society of America* 29: 98–104.

Ladefoged, P., J. De Clerk, M. Lindau, and G. Papcun. 1972. An auditory-motor theory of speech production. *UCLA Working Papers in Phonetics* 22: 48–76.

Laitman, J. T., and R. C. Heimbuch. 1982. The basicranium of Plio-Pleistocene hominids as an indicator of their upper respiratory systems. *American Journal of Physical Anthropology* 59: 323–344.

Laitman, J. T., R. C. Heimbuch, and E. S. Crelin. 1979. The basicranium of fossil hominids as an indicator of their upper respiratory systems. *American Journal of Physical Anthropology* 51: 15–34.

Lange, K. W., T. W. Robbins, C. D. Marsden, M. James, A. M. Owen, and G. M. Paul. 1992. L-dopa withdrawal in Parkinson's disease selectively impairs cognitive performance in tests sensitive to frontal lobe dysfunction. *Psychopharmacology* 107: 394–404.

Laplane, D., M. Baulac, and D. Widlocher. 1984. Pure psychic akinesia with bilateral lesions of basal ganglia. *Journal of Neurology, Neurosurgery, and Psychiatry* 47: 377–385.

Lashley, K. S. 1951. The problem of serial order in behavior. In *Cerebral mechanisms in behavior,* ed. L. A. Jefress. New York: Wiley. Pp. 112–146.

Leakey, M. G., C. S. Feibel, I. McDougall, and A. Walker. 1995. New four-million-year-old hominid species from Kanapoi and Allia Bay, Kenya. *Nature* 376: 565–571.

Leiner, H. C., A. L. Leiner, and R. S. Dow. 1991. The human cerebro-cerebellar system: Its computing, cognitive, and language skills. *Behavioral Brain Research* 44: 113–128.

———1993. Cognitive and language functions of the human cerebellum. *Trends in Neuroscience* 16: 444–447, 453–454.

Leonard, L. E. 1998. *Children with specific language impairment.* Cambridge, Mass.: MIT Press.

Levelt, W. J. 1989. *Speaking: From intention to articulation.* Cambridge, Mass.: MIT Press.

Liberman, A. M., F. S. Cooper, D. P. Shankweiler, and M. Studdert-Kennedy. 1967. Perception of the speech code. *Psychological Review* 74: 431–461.

Liberman, A. M., and I. G. Mattingly. 1985. The motor theory of speech perception revised. *Cognition* 21: 1–36.

Liberman, F. Z. 1979. Learning by neural nets. Ph.D diss., Brown University.

Lichtheim, L. 1885. On aphasia. *Brain* 7: 433–484.

Lieberman, D. E. 1995. Testing hypotheses about recent human evolution from skulls. *Current Anthropology* 36: 159–198.

———1998. Sphenoid shortening and the evolution of modern human cranial shape. *Nature* 393: 158–162.

Lieberman, D. E., and R. C. McCarthy. 1999. The ontogeny of cranial base angulation in humans and chimpanzees and its implications for reconstructing pharyngeal dimensions. *Journal of Human Evolution* 36: 487–517.

Lieberman, M. R., and P. Lieberman. 1973. Olson's "projective verse" and the use of breath control as a structural element. *Language and Style* 5: 287–298.

Lieberman, P. 1961. Perturbations in vocal pitch. *Journal of the Acoustical Society of America* 33: 597–603.

———1963. Some measures of the fundamental periodicity of normal and pathologic larynges. Journal of the Acoustical Society of America 35: 344–353.

———1967. *Intonation, perception, and language.* Cambridge, Mass.: MIT Press.

———1968. Primate vocalizations and human linguistic ability. *Journal of the Acoustical Society of America* 44: 1157–64.

———1973. On the evolution of human language: A unified view. *Cognition* 2: 59–64.

———1975. *On the origins of language: An introduction to the evolution of speech.* New York: Macmillan.

———1980. On the development of vowel production in young children. In *Child phonology, perception, and production,* ed. G. Yeni-Komshian and J. Kavanagh. New York: Academic Press. Pp. 113–142.

———1984. *The biology and evolution of language.* Cambridge, Mass.: Harvard University Press.

———1985. On the evolution of human syntactic ability: Its pre-adaptive bases—motor control and speech. *Journal of Human Evolution* 14: 657–668.

———1991. *Uniquely human: The evolution of speech, thought, and selfless behavior.* Cambridge, Mass.: Harvard University Press.

———1992. Could an autonomous syntax module have evolved? *Brain and Language* 43: 768–774.

———1994a. Biologically bound behavior, free will, and human evolution. In *Conflict and cooperation in nature,* ed. J. I. Casti. New York: Wiley. Pp. 133–163.

———1994b. Hyoid bone position and speech: Reply to Arensburg et al. (1990). *American Journal of Physical Anthropology* 94: 275–278.

———1994c. Functional tongues and Neanderthal vocal tract reconstruction: A reply to Houghton (1993). *American Journal of Physical Anthropology* 95: 443–452.

———1998. *Eve spoke: Human language and human evolution.* New York: W. W. Norton.

Lieberman, P., and S. E. Blumstein. 1988. *Speech physiology, speech perception, and acoustic phonetics.* Cambridge: Cambridge University Press.

Lieberman, P., E. S. Crelin, and D. H. Klatt. 1972. Phonetic ability and related anatomy of the newborn, adult human, Neanderthal man, and the chimpanzee. *American Anthropologist* 74: 287–307.

Lieberman, P., L. S. Feldman, S. Aronson, and B. Engen. 1989. Sentence comprehension, syntax, and vowel duration in aged people. *Clinical Linguistics and Phonetics* 3: 299–311.

Lieberman, P., J. Friedman, and L. S. Feldman. 1990. Syntactic deficits in Parkinson's disease. *Journal of Nervous and Mental Disease* 178: 360–365.

Lieberman, P., E. T. Kako, J. Friedman, G. Tajchman, L. S. Feldman and E. B. Jiminez. 1992. Speech production, syntax comprehension, and cognitive deficits in Parkinson's disease. *Brain and Language* 43: 169–189.

Lieberman, P., B. G. Kanki, and A. Protopapas. 1995. Speech production and cognitive decrements on Mount Everest. *Aviation, Space, and Environmental Medicine* 66: 857–864.

Lieberman, P., B. G. Kanki, A. Protopapas, E. Reed, and J. W. Youngs. 1994. Cognitive defects at altitude. *Nature* 372: 325.

Lieberman, P., W. Katz, A. Jongman, R. Zimmerman, and M. Miller. 1984. Measures of the sentence intonation of read and spontaneous speech in American English. *Journal of the Acoustical Society of America* 77: 649–657.

Lieberman, P., R. H. Meskill, M. Chatillon, and H. Schupack. 1985. Phonetic speech deficits in dyslexia. *Journal of Speech and Hearing Research* 28: 480–486.

Lieberman, P., and C.-Y. Tseng. 1994. Subcortical pathways essential for speech, language, and cognition: Implications for hominid evolution. *American Journal of Physical Anthropology* 93 (suppl. 16): 130.

———In preparation. Some speech production and syntax comprehension deficits of Parkinson's disease in Chinese-speaking subjects.

Lindblom, B. 1988. Models of phonetic variation and selection. *Language change and biological evolution.* Turin, Italy: Institute for Scientific Interchange.

———1996. Role of articulation in speech perception: Clues from production. *Journal of the Acoustical Society of America* 99: 1683–92.

Linebarger, M., M. Schwartz, and E. Saffran. 1983. Sensitivity to grammatical structure in so-called agrammatic aphasics. *Cognition* 13: 361–392.

Lisker, L., and A. S. Abramson. 1964. A cross-language study of voicing in initial stops: Acoustical measurements. *Word* 20: 384–442.

Longoni, A. M., J. T. E. Richardson, and A. Aiello. 1993. Articulatory rehearsal and phonological storage in working memory. *Memory and Cognition* 21: 11–22.

Lubker, J., and T. Gay. 1982. Anticipatory labial coarticulation: Experimental, biological, and linguistic variables. *Journal of the Acoustical Society of America* 71: 437–438.

MacDonald, M. C. 1994. Probabilistic constraints and syntactic ambiguity resolution. *Language and Cognitive Processes* 9: 157–201.

MacDonald, M. C., N. J. Perlmutter, and M. S. Seidenberg. 1994. Lexical nature of syntactic ambiguity resolution. *Psychological Review* 101: 676–703.

MacLean, P. D. 1973. A triune concept of the brain and behavior. In *The Hincks Memorial Lectures,* ed. T. Boag and D. Campbell. Toronto: University of Toronto Press. Pp. 6–66.

MacLean, P. D., and J. D. Newman. 1988. Role of midline frontolimbic cortex in the production of the isolation call of squirrel monkeys. *Brain Research* 450: 111–123.

MacNeilage, P. F. 1987. The evolution of hemispheric specialization for manual function and language. In *Higher brain functions: Recent explorations of the brain's emergent properties,* ed. S. P. Wise. New York: John Wiley & Sons.

MacNeill, D. 1985. So you think gestures are nonverbal? *Psychological Review* 92: 350–371.

MacWhinney, B. 1991. Implementations are not conceptualizations: Revising the verb-learning model. *Cognition* 40: 121–157.

Magee, J. C., and D. Johnston. 1997. A synaptically controlled, associative signal for Hebbian plasticity in hippocampal neurons. *Science* 275: 209–213.

Malapani, C., B. Pillon, B. Dubois, and Y. Agid. 1994. Impaired simultaneous cognitive task performance in Parkinson's disease: A dopamine-related dysfunction. *Neurology* 44: 319–326.

Manley, R. S., and L. C. Braley. 1950. Masticatory performance and efficiency. *Journal of Dental Research* 29: 314–321.

Manley, R. S., and F. R. Shiere. 1950. The effect of dental efficiency on mastication and food preference. *Oral Surgery, Oral Medicine, and Oral Pathology* 3: 674–685.

Marie, P. 1926 *Traveaux et mémoires.* Paris: Masson.

Marin, O., W. J. A. J. Smeets, and A. Gonzalez. 1998. Evolution of the basal ganlia in tetrapods: A new perspective based on recent studies in amphibians. *Trends in Neuroscience* 21: 487–494.

Markram, H., J. Lubke, M. Frotscher, and B. Sakmann. 1997. Regulation of synaptic efficacy by coincidence of postsynaptic APs and EPSRs. *Science* 275: 213–215.

Marsden, C. D., and J. A. Obeso. 1994. The functions of the basal ganglia and the paradox of stereotaxic surgery in Parkinson's disease. *Brain* 117: 877–897.

Martin, A., J. V. Haxby, F. M. Lalonde, C. L. Wiggs, and L. G. Ungerleider. 1995. Discrete cortical regions associated with knowledge of color and knowledge of action. *Science* 270: 102–105.

Martin, A., C. L. Wiggs, L. G. Ungerleider, and J. V. Haxby. 1995. Neural correlates of category-specific knowledge. *Nature* 379: 649–652.

Massaro, D. W., and M. M. Cohen. 1995. Perceiving talking faces. *Current Directions in Psychological Science* 4: 104–109.

Mayr, E. 1982. *The growth of biological thought.* Cambridge, Mass.: Harvard University Press.

McCowan, T. D., and A. Keith. 1939. *The stone age of Mount Carmel.* Vol. 2: *The fossil human remains from the Levalloisio-Mousterian.* Oxford: Clarendon Press.

McGrew, W. C. 1993. The intelligent use of tools: Twenty propositions. In *Tools, language, and cognition in human evolution,* ed. K. R. Gibson and T. Ingold. Cambridge: Cambridge University Press. Pp. 151–170.

McGurk, H., and J. MacDonald. 1976. Hearing lips and seeing voices. *Nature* 263: 747–748.

Mega, M. S., and M. F. Alexander. 1994. Subcortical aphasia: The core profile of capsulostriatal infarction. *Neurology* 44: 1824–29.

Mellars, P. 1996. *The Neanderthal legacy: An archaeological perspective from Western Europe.* Princeton: Princeton University Press.

Mentzel, H. J., C. Gaser, H. P. Volz, R. Rzanny, F. Hager, H. Aauer, and W. A. Kaiser. 1998. Cognitive stimulation with the Wisconsin Card Sorting Test: Functional MR imaging at 1.5 T. *Radiology* 207: 399–404.

Merzenich, M. M. 1987. Cerebral cortex: A quiet revolution in thinking. *Nature* 328: 572–573.

Merzenich, M. M., R. Nelson, M. Stryker, M. Cynader, A. Schoppmann, and J. Zook. 1984. Somatosensory cortical map changes following digit amputation in adult monkeys. *Journal of Comparative Neurology* 224: 591–605.

Mesulam, M. M. 1985. Patterns in behavioral neuroanatomy: Association areas, the limbic system, and hemispheric specialization. In *Principles of behavioral neurology,* ed. M. M. Mesulam. Philadelphia: F. A. Davis. Pp. 1–70.

———1990. Large-scale neurocognitive networks and distributed processing for attention, language, and memory. *Annals of Neurology* 28: 597–613.

Metter, E. J., D. Kempler, C. A. Jackson, W. R. Hanson, J. C. Mazziotta, and M. E. Phelps. 1989. Cerebral glucose metabolism in Wernicke's, Broca's, and conduction aphasia. *Archives of Neurology* 46: 27–34.

Metter, E. J., D. Kempler, C. A. Jackson, W. R. Hanson, W. H. Reige, L. M. Camras, J. C. Mazziotta, and M. E. Phelps. 1987. Cerebular glucose metabolism in chronic aphasia. *Neurology* 37: 1599–1606.

Metter, E. J., W. H. Riege, W. R. Hanson, M. E. Phelps, and D. E. Kuhl. 1984. Local cerebral metabolic rates of glucose in movement and language disorders from positron tomography. *American Journal of Physiology* 246: R897–R900.

Miceli, G., A. Mazzucchi, L. Menn, and H. Goodglass. 1983. Contrasting cases of Italian agrammatic aphasia without comprehension disorder. *Brain and Language* 19: 65–97.

Middleton, F. A., and P. L. Strick. 1994. Anatomical evidence for cerebellar and basal ganglia involvement in higher cognition. *Science* 266: 458–461.

Milberg, W., S. E. Blumstein, and B. Dworetzky. 1987. Processing of lexical ambiguities in aphasia. *Brain and Language* 31: 138–150.

———1988. Phonological processing and lexical access in aphasia. *Brain and Language* 34: 279–293.

Miles, C., D. M. Jones, and C. A. Madden. 1991. Locus of the irrelevant speech effect in short-term memory. *Journal of Experimental Psychology: Learning, Memory, and Cognition* 17: 578–584.

Miller, G. A. 1956. The magical number seven, plus or minus two: Some limits on our capacity for processing information. *Psychological Review* 63: 81–97.

———1963. Some psychological studies of grammar. *American Psychologist* 17: 748–762.

Miller, J. L., K. P. Green, and A. Reeves. 1986. Effect of speaking rate on voice-onset time. *Phonetica* 43: 106–115.

Mirenowicz, J., and W. Schultz. 1996. Preferential activation of midbrain dopamine neurons by appetitive rather than aversive stimuli. *Nature* 379: 449–451.

Miyai, I., A. D. Blau, M. J. Reding, and B. T. Volpe. 1997. Patients with stroke confined to basal ganglia have diminished response to rehabilitation efforts. *Neurology* 48: 95–101.

Morris, R. G., J. J. Downes, B. J. Sahakian, J. L. Evenden, A. Heald, and T. W. Robbins. 1988. Planning and spatial working memory in Parkinson's disease. *Journal of Neurology, Neurosurgery, and Psychiatry* 51: 757–766.

Müller, J. 1848. *The physiology of the senses, voice, and muscular motion with the mental faculties.* Trans. W. Baly. London: Walton and Maberly.

Naeser, M. A., M. P. Alexander, N. Helms-Estabrooks, H. L. Levine, S. A. Laughlin, and N. Geschwind. 1982. Aphasia with predominantly subcortical lesion sites: Description of three capsular/putaminal aphasia syndromes. *Archives of Neurology* 39: 2–14.

Nakano, H., J. Hochstadt, and P. Lieberman. In preparation. Sentence comprehension in Parkinson's disease: Deficits in verbal working memory and sequencing.

Natsopoulos, D., G. Grouios, S. Bostantzopoulou, G. Mentenopoulos, Z. Katsarou, and J. Logothetis. 1993. Algorithmic and heuristic strategies in comprehension of complement clauses by patients with Parkinson's disease. *Neuropsychologia* 31: 951–964

Nearey, T. 1979. *Phonetic features for vowels.* Bloomington: Indiana University Linguistics Club.

Negus, V. E. 1949. *The comparative anatomy and physiology of the larynx.* New York: Hafner.

Nelson, T. O., J. Dunlosky, D. M. White, J. Steinberg, B. D. Townes, and D. Anderson. 1990. Cognition and metacognition at extreme altitudes on Mount Everest. *Journal of Experimental Psychology: General* 119: 367–374.

Nelson, T. O., and B. Kanki. 1989. Effects of altitude on metacognition and on the retrieval of information from memory at Mount Everest. *Nasa–Ames University Consortium Final Report.* Ames, Calif.

Nespoulous, J.-L., M. Dordain, C. Perron, B. Ska, D. Bub, D. Caplan, J. Mehler, and A. R. Lecours. 1988. Agrammatism in sentence production without comprehension deficits: Reduced availability of syntactic structures and/or grammatical morphemes: A case study. *Brain and Language* 33: 273–295.

Newman, J. D., and P. D. Maclean. 1982. Effects of tegmental lesions on the isolation call of squirrel monkeys. *Brain Research* 232: 317–329.

Newmeyer, F. 1991. Functional explanation in linguistics and the origin of language. *Language and Communication* 11: 3–28.

Nisimura, H., K. Hashikawa, K. Doi, T. Iwaki, Y. Watanabe, H. Kusuoka, T. Nishimura, and T. Kubo. 1999. Sign language "heard" in the auditory cortex. *Nature* 397: 116.

Nottebohm, F. 1984. Vocal learning and its possible relation to replaceable synapses and neurons. In *Biological perspectives on language,* ed. D. Caplan, A. R. Lecours, and A. Smith. Cambridge, Mass.: MIT Press. Pp. 65–95.

Nottebohm, F., and M. E. Nottebohm. 1976. Left hypoglossal dominance in the control of Canary and White-Crowned Sparrow song. *Journal of Comparative Physiology: Sensory, Neural, and Behavioral Physiology* 108: 171–192.

Nudo, R. J., G. W. Milliken, W. M. Jenkins, and M. M. Merzenich. 1996. Use-dependent alterations of movement representations in primary motor cortex of adult squirrel monkeys. *Journal of Neuroscience* 16: 785–807.

Ohala, J. 1970. *Aspects of the control and production of speech.* UCLA Working Papers in Phonetics, no. 15. Los Angeles: UCLA Phonetics Laboratory.

Ojemann, G. A., and C. Mateer. 1979. Human language cortex: Localization of memory, syntax, and sequential motor-phoneme identification systems. *Science* 205: 1401–03.

Ojemann, G. A., F. Ojemann, E. Lettich, and M. Berger. 1989. Cortical language localization in left dominant hemisphere: An electrical stimulation mapping investigation in 117 patients. *Journal of Neurosurgery* 71: 316–326.

Olmsted, D. L. 1971. *Out of the mouths of babes.* The Hague: Mouton.

Owren, M. J. 1990. Acoustic classification of alarm calls by vervet monkeys (*Cercopithecus aethiops*) and humans. II: Synthetic calls. *Journal of Comparative Psychology* 104: 29–40.

Owren, M. J., and R. Bernacki. 1988. The acoustic features of vervet monkey (*Cercopithecus aethiops*) alarm calls. *Journal of the Acoustical Society of America* 83: 1927–35.

Palmer, J. B., and K. M. Hiiemae. 1998. Integration of oral and pharyngeal bolus propulsion: A new model for the physiology of swallowing. *Journal of Diet, Eating, and Swallowing Rehabilitation* (Japan) 1: 15–30.

Palmer, J. B., K. M. Hiiemae, and J. Liu. 1997. Tongue-jaw linkages in human feeding: A preliminary videofluorographic study. *Archives of Oral Biology* 6: 429–441.

Pantev, C., R. Oostenveld, A. Engelien, B. Ross, L. E. Roberts, and M. Hoke. 1998. Increased auditory cortical representation in musicians. *Nature* 392: 811–818.

Parent, A. 1986. *Comparative neurobiology of the basal ganglia.* New York: John Wiley.

Parkinson's Study Group. 1989. The DATATOP series. *Archives of Neurology* 46: 1052–60.

Pascual-Leone, A., D. Nguyet, L. G. Cohen, J. P. Brasil-Neto, A. Cammaroya, and M. Hallet. 1995. Modulation of motor responses evoked by transcranial magnetic stimulation during the acquisition of new fine motor skills. *Journal of Neurophysiology* 74: 1037–1045.

Passingham, R. E. 1985. Prefrontal cortex and sequencing of movements in monkeys (*Macaca mulatta*). *Neuropsychologia* 23: 453–462.

Paterson, A. H., Lin Yann-Rong, Li Zhijang, K. F. Schertz, J. F. Doebley, S. R. M. Pinson, Liu Sin-Chieh, J. W. Stansel, and J. E. Irvine. 1995. Convergent domestication of cereal crops by independent mutations at corresponding genetic loci. *Science* 269: 1714–17.

Patterson, D. K., and I. M. Pepperberg. 1994. A comparative study of human and parrot phonation: Acoustic and articulatory correlates of vowels. *Journal of the Acoustical Society of America* 96: 634–648.

Paulesu, E., C. Firth, and R. Frackowiak. 1993. The neural correlates of the verbal component of working memory. *Nature* 362: 342–345.

Paus, T., D. W. Perry, R. A. Zatorre, K. J. Worsley, and A. C. Evans. 1996. Modulation of cerebral blood flow in the human auditory cortex during speech: Role of motor-to-sensory discharges. *European Journal of Neuroscience* 8: 2236–46.

Pennisi, E. 1996. Evolutionary and systematic biologists converge. *Science* 273: 181–182.

Pepperberg, I. M. 1981. Functional vocalizations by an African Grey Parrot (*Psittacus erithacus*). *Zeitschrift für Tierpsychologie* 55: 139–160.

Percheron, G., and M. Fillon. 1991. Parallel processing in the basal ganglia up to a point. *Trends in Neuroscience* 14: 55–59.

Percheron, G., J. Yelnick, and C. A. Francois. 1984. Golgi analysis of the primate globus pallidus. III: Spatial organization of the striato-pallidal complex. *Journal of Comparative Neurology* 227: 214–227.

Perkell, J. S. 1969. *Physiology of speech production: Results and implications of a quantitative cineradiographic study.* Cambridge, Mass.: MIT Press.

Perkell, J. S., and W. L. Nelson. 1982. Articulatory targets and speech motor control: A study of vowel production. In *Speech motor control*, ed. S. Grillner, A. Persson, B. Lindblom, and J. Lubker. New York: Pergamon. Pp. 187–204.

———1985. Variability in the production of the vowels /i/, /u/, and /a/. *Journal of the Acoustical Society of America* 77: 1889–95.

Perrault, C. 1676. *Mémoires pour servir à l'histoire naturelle des animaux.* Paris: L'Imprimerie Royale.

Peterson, G. E., and H. L. Barney. 1952. Control methods used in a study of the vowels. *Journal of the Acoustical Society of America* 24: 175–184.

Peterson, S. E., and J. A. Fiez. 1993. The processing of single words studied with positron emission tomography. *Annual Review of Neuroscience* 16: 509–530.

Peterson, S. E., P. T. Fox, M. I. Posner, M. Mintun, and M. E. Raichle. 1988. Positron emission tomographic studies of the cortical anatomy of single-word processing. *Nature* 331: 585–589.

Phillips, J. G., E. Chiu, J. L. Bradshaw, and R. Iansek. 1995. Impaired movement sequencing in patients with Huntington's disease: A kinematic analysis. *Neuropsychologia* 33: 365–369.

Piatelli-Palmarini, M. 1989. Evolution, selection, and cognition: From "learning" to parameter-setting in biology and the study of language. *Cognition* 31: 1–44.

Pickett, E. R. 1998. Language and the cerebellum. Ph.D. diss., Brown University.

Pickett, E. R., Kuniholm, A. Protopapas, J. Friedman, and P. Lieberman. 1998. Selective speech motor, syntax, and cognitive deficits associated with bilateral damage to the head of the caudate nucleus and the putamen: A single case study. *Neuropsychologia* 36: 173–188.

Pierce, J. D. 1985. A review of attempts to condition operantly Alloprimate vocalizations. *Primates* 26: 202–213.

Pinker, S. 1994. *The language instinct: How the mind creates language.* New York: William Morrow.

———1998. *How the mind works.* New York: W. W. Norton.

Pinker, S., and P. Bloom. 1990. Natural selection and natural language. *Behavioral and Brain Sciences* 13: 707–784.

Pinker, S., and A. Prince. 1988. On language and connectionism: An analysis of a parallel distributed processing model of language acquisition. *Cognition* 28: 73–193.

Pitt, M. A., and A. G. Samuel. 1995. Lexical and sublexical feedback in auditory word recognition. *Cognitive Psychology* 29: 149–188.

Plomin, R. 1989. Environment and genes: Determinants of behavior. *American Psychologist* 44: 105–111.

Pollack, I., and J. M. Pickett. 1963. The intelligibility of excerpts from conversation. *Language and Speech* 6: 165–171.

Premack, D. 1972. Language in chimpanzee? *Science* 172: 808–822.

Rauschecker, J. P., and M. Korte. 1993. Auditory compensation for early blindness in cat cerebral cortex. *Journal of Neuroscience* 18: 4538–48.

Raymond, J. L., S. G. Lisberger, and M. D. Mauk. 1996. The cerebellum: A neuronal learning machine? *Science* 272: 1126–31.

Remez, R. E., P. E. Rubin, D. B. Pisoni, and T. O. Carrell. 1981. Speech perception without traditional cues. *Science* 212: 947–950.

Rizzolatti, G., and M. A. Arbib. 1998. Language within our grasp. *Trends in Neuroscience* 21: 188–194.

Rizzolatti, G., L. Fadiga, V. Galiese, and L. Fogassi. 1996. Premotor cortex and the recognition of motor actions. *Cognitive Brain Research* 3: 131–141.

Rothlind, J. C., F. W. Bylsma, C. Peyser, S. E. Folstein, and J. Brandt. 1993. Cognitive and motor correlates of everyday functioning in early Huntington's disease. *Journal of Nervous and Mental Disease* 181: 194–199.

Ruhlen, M. *On the origin of language: Tracing the evolution of the mother tongue.* New York: John Wiley.

Rumbaugh, D. M., and E. S. Savage-Rumbaugh. 1992. Biobehavioral roots of language: Words, apes, and a child. Conference paper presented at University of Bielefeld, Germany.

Rumelhart, D. E., J. L. McClelland, and the PDP Research Group. 1986. *Parallel distributed processing.* Vol. 1: *Explorations in the microstructures of cognition.* Cambridge, Mass.: MIT Press.

Russell, G. O. 1928. *The vowel.* Columbus: Ohio State University Press.

Ryalls, J. 1981. Motor aphasia: Acoustic correlates of phonetic disintegration in vowels. *Neuropsychologia* 20: 355–360.

———1986. An acoustic study of vowel production in aphasia. *Brain and Language* 29: 48–67.

Sachs, J., P. Lieberman, and D. Erikson. 1973. Anatomical and cultural determinants of male and female speech. In *Language attitudes: Current trends and prospects. Monograph No. 25,* ed. R. W. Shuy and R. W. Fasold. Washington, D.C.: Georgetown University.

Sadato, N., A. Pascual-Leone, J. Grafman, V. Ibanez, M.-P. Delber, G. Dold, and M.

Hallet. 1996. Activation of the primary visual cortex by Braille reading in blind subjects. *Nature* 380: 525–528.

Saffran, J. R., R. N. Aslin, and E. L. Newport. Statistical learning by 8-month-old infants. *Science* 274: 1926–28.

Sanes, J. N., and J. P. Donoghue. 1996. Static and dynamic organization of motor cortex. *Advances in Neurology, Brain Plasticity* 73: 277–296.

———1997. Dynamic motor cortical organization. *The Neuroscientist* 3: 158–165.

———In press. Plasticity of cortical representations and its implication for neurorehabilitation. In *Principles and practice of rehabilitation medicine,* ed. B. T. Dhanai. Baltimore: Williams and Wilkins.

Sanes, J. N., J. P. Donoghue, Venkatesan Thangaraj, R. R. Edelman, and S. Warach. 1995. Shared neural substrates controlling hand movements in human motor cortex. *Science* 268: 1775–77.

Sarich, V. M. 1974. Just how old is the hominid line? In *Yearbook of physical anthropology, 1973.* Washington, D.C.: American Association of Physical Anthropologists.

Saussure, F. de. 1959. *Course in general linguistics.* Trans. W. Baskin. New York: McGraw-Hill.

Savage-Rumbaugh, E. S., K. McDonald, R. A. Sevcik, W. D. Hopkins, and E. Rubert. 1986. Spontaneous symbol acquisition and communicative use by pygmy chimpanzees *(Pan paniscus). Journal of Experimental Psychology: General* 115: 211–235.

Savage-Rumbaugh, E. S., and D. Rumbaugh. 1993. The emergence of language. In *Tools, language, and cognition in human evolution,* ed. K. R. Gibson and T. Ingold. Cambridge: Cambridge University Press. Pp. 86–100.

Savin, H. L., and E. Perchonok. 1965. Grammatical structure and the immediate recall of English sentences. *Journal of Verbal Learning and Verbal Behavior* 4: 348–353.

Schepartz, L. A. 1993. Language and modern human origins. *Yearbook of Physical Anthropology* 36: 91–126.

Schluter, D. 1994. Experimental evidence that competition promotes divergence in adaptive radiation. *Science* 266: 798–801.

Schmahmann, J. D. 1991. An emerging concept: The cerebellar contribution to higher function. *Archives of Neurology* 48: 1178–86.

Seebach, B. S., N. Intrator, P. Lieberman, and L. N. Cooper. 1994. A model of prenatal acquisition of speech parameters. *Proceedings of the National Academy of Sciences, USA* 91: 7473–76.

Sejnowski, T. 1997. The year of the dendrite. *Science* 275: 178–179.

Semaw, S., P. Renne, J. W. K. Harris, C. S. Feibel, R. L. Bernor, N. Fesseha, and K. Mowbray. 1997. 2.5-million-year-old stone tools from Gona, Ethiopia. *Science* 385: 333–336.

Semendeferi, K., H. Damasio, R. Frank, and G. W. Van Hoesen. 1997. The evolution of the frontal lobes: A volumetric analysis based on three-dimensional reconstructions of magnetic resonance scans of human and ape brains. *Journal of Human Evolution* 32: 375–378.

Sereno, J., S. R. Baum, G. C. Marean, and P. Lieberman. 1987. Acoustic analyses and perceptual data on anticipatory labial coarticulation in adults and children. *Journal of the Acoustical Society of America* 81: 512–519.

Sereno, J., and P. Lieberman. 1987. Developmental aspects of lingual coarticulation. *Journal of Phonetics* 15: 247–257.

Shallice, T., and B. Butterworth. 1977. Short-term memory and spontaneous speech. *Neuropsychologia* 15: 729–735.

Shankweiler, D., S. Crain, P. Gorell, and B. Tuller. 1989. Reception of language in Broca's aphasia. *Language and Cognitive Processes* 4: 1–33.

Shea, J. J. 1998. Neanderthal and early modern human behavioral variability: A regional-scale approach to lithic evidence for hunting in the Levantine Moustarian. *Current Anthropology* 39 (suppl.): 45–78.

Singer, W. 1995. Development and plasticity of cortical processing architectures. *Science* 270: 758–769.

Singleton, J. L., and E. L. Newport. 1989. When learners surpass their models: The acquisition of American Sign Language from impoverished input. In *Proceedings of the 14th Annual Boston University Conference on Language Development.* Vol. 15. Boston: Boston University, Program in Applied Linguistics.

Slobin, D. L. 1991. Aphasia in Turkish: Speech production in Broca's and Wernicke's patients. *Brain and Language* 41: 149–164.

Smith, B. L. 1978. Temporal aspects of English speech production: A developmental perspective. *Journal of Phonetics* 6: 37–68.

Smith, B. L., J. Wasowicz, and J. Preston. 1986. Durational characteristics of the speech of normal elderly adults. Paper presented at the annual meeting of the Acoustical Society of America, Anaheim, Calif.

Spurzheim, J. K. 1815. *The physiognomical system of Gall and Spurzheim.* London.

Stephan, H., H. Frahm, and G. Baron. 1981. New and revised data on volumes of brain structures in insectivores and primates. *Folia Primatologia* 35: 1–29.

Stevens, K. N. 1972. Quantal nature of speech. In *Human communication: A unified view,* ed. E. E. David Jr. and P. B. Denes. New York: McGraw-Hill.

Stevens, K. N., and A. S. House. 1955. Development of a quantitative description of vowel articulation. *Journal of the Acoustical Society of America* 27: 484–493.

Stokoe, W. 1978. Sign language versus spoken language. *Sign Language Studies* 18: 69–90.

Story, B. H., I. R. Titze, and E. A. Hoffman. 1996. Vocal tract area functions from magnetic resonance imaging. *Journal of the Acoustical Society of America* 100: 537–554.

Stringer, C. B. 1992. Evolution of early humans. In *The Cambridge encyclopedia of human evolution,* ed. S. Jones, R. Martin, and D. Pilbeam. Cambridge: Cambridge University Press. Pp. 241–251.

Stringer, C. B., and P. Andrews. 1988. Genetic and fossil evidence for the origin of modern humans. *Science* 239: 1263–68.

Stromswold, K., D. Caplan, N. Alpert, and S. Rausch. 1996. Localization of syntactic processing by positron emission tomography. *Brain and Language* 51: 452–473.

Strub, R. L. 1989. Frontal lobe syndrome on a patient with bilateral globus pallidus lesions. *Archives of Neurology* 46: 1024–27.

Stuss, D. T., and D. F. Benson. 1986. *The frontal lobes.* New York: Raven Press.

Susman, R. L. 1994. Fossil evidence for early hominid tool use. *Science* 265: 1570–73.

Sutton, D., and U. Jurgens. 1988. Neural control of vocalization. In *Comparative primate biology,* ed. H. D. Steklis and J. Erwin. Vol. 4, pp. 625–647. New York: Arthur D. Liss.

Tallal, P. 1976. Rapid auditory processing in normal and disordered language development. *Journal of Speech and Hearing Research* 19: 561–571.

Taylor, A. E., J. A. Saint-Cyr, and A. E. Lang. 1986. Frontal lobe dysfunction in Parkinson's disease. *Brain* 109: 845–883.

———1990. Memory and learning in early Parkinson's disease: Evidence for a "frontal lobe syndrome." *Brain and Cognition* 13: 211–232.

Terrace, H. S., L. A. Petitto, R. J. Sanders, and T. G. Bever. 1979. Can an ape create a sentence? *Science* 206: 821–901.

Thatch, W. T., J. W. Mink, H. P. Goodkin, and J. G. Keating. 1993. Combining versus gating motor programs: Differential roles for cerebellum and basal ganglia. In *Role of the cerebellum and basal ganglia in voluntary movement,* ed. N. Mano, I. Hmada, and M. R. DeLong. Amsterdam: Elsevier.

Thelen, E. 1984, Learning to walk: Ecological demands and phylogenetic constraints. In *Advances in infancy research,* ed. L. Lipsitt. Vol. 3, pp. 213–250. Norwood, N.J: Ablex.

Thieme, H. 1997. Lower Paleolithic hunting spears from Germany. *Nature* 385: 807–810.

Tishkoff, S. A., E. Dietzsch, W. Speed, A. J. Pakstis, J. R. Kidd, K. Cheung, B. Bonne-Tamir, A. S. Santachiara-Benerecetti, P. Moral, M. Krings, S. Paabo, E. Watson, N. Risch, T. Jenkins, and K. K. Kidd. 1996. Global patterns of linkage disequilibrium at the CD4 locus and modern human origins. *Science* 271: 1380–87.

Tooby, J., and L. Cosmides. 1992. Psychological foundations of culture. In *Psychological foundations of culture,* ed. J. Barkow, L. Cosmides, and J. Tooby. New York: Oxford University Press. Pp. 19–136.

Toth, N., and K. Schick. 1993. Early stone industries. In *Tools, language, and cognition in human evolution,* ed. K. R. Gibson and T. Ingold. Cambridge: Cambridge University Press. Pp. 346–362.

Tseng, C.-Y. 1981. An acoustic study of tones in Mandarin. Ph.D. diss., Brown University.

Tyson, E. 1699. *Oran-outang, sive homo sylvestrus; or the anatomie of a pygmie compared with that of a monkey, an ape, and a man.* London: Thomas Bennet and Daniel Brown.

Umeda, N. 1975. Vowel duration in American English. *Journal of the Acoustical Society of America* 58: 434–446.

Ungerleider, L. G. 1995. Functional brain imaging studies of cortical mechanisms for memory. *Science* 270: 769–775.

Vallar, G., A. M. D. Betta, and M. C. Silveri. 1997. The phonological short-term store-rehearsal system. *Neuropsychologia* 35: 795–812.

Vandermeersch, B. 1981. *Les hommes fossiles de Qafzeh, Israel.* Paris: CNRS.

Vargha-Khadem, F., K. E. Watkins, R. Passingham, and P. Fletcher. 1995. Cognitive and praxic deficits in a large family with a genetically transmitted speech and language disorder. *Proceedings of the National Academy of Sciences* 92: 930–933.

Vargha-Khadem, F., K. E. Watkins, C. J. Price, J. Ashbruner, K. J. Alcock, A. Connelly, R. S. J. Frackowiak, K. J. Friston, M. E. Pembrey, M. Mishkin, D. G. Gadian, and R. E. Passingham. 1998. Neural basis of an inherited speech and language disorder. *Proceedings of the National Academy of Sciences* 95: 2695–2700.

Vleck, E. 1970. Etude comparative onto-phylogénétique de l'enfant du Pech-de-L'Aze par rapport à d'autres enfants neanderthaliens. In *L'enfant Pech-de-L'Aze,* ed. D. Feremback. Paris: Masson. Pp. 149–186.

Walker, A. E. 1940. *Journal of Comparative Neurology* 73: 59–62.

Walker, A., and P. Shipman. 1996. *The wisdom of the bones.* New York: Alfred A. Knopf.

Wallesch, C.-W., and R. A. Fehrenbach. 1988. On the neurolinguistic nature of language abnormalities in Huntington's disease. *Journal of Neurology, Neurosurgery, and Psychiatry* 51: 367–373.

Warden, C. J., and L. H. Warner. 1928. The sensory capacities and intelligence of dogs, with a report on the ability of the noted dog "Fellow" to respond to verbal stimuli. *Quarterly Review of Biology* 3: 1–28.

Warrington, E., V. Logue, and R. Pratt. 1971. The anatomical localization of the selective impairment of auditory verbal short-term memory. *Neuropsychologia* 9: 377–387.

Wechsler, D. 1944. *Measurement of adult intelligence.* Baltimore: Williams and Wilkins.

Wernicke, C. 1874. The aphasic symptom complex: A psychological study on a neurological basis. Breslau: Kohn and Weigert. Reprinted in *Boston studies in the philosophy of science,* vol. 4, ed. R. S. Cohen and M. W. Wartofsky. Boston: Reidel.

White, T. D., G. Suwu, and B. Asfaw. 1994. *Australopithecus ramidus,* a new species of early hominid from Aramis, Ethiopia. *Nature* 371: 306–312.

Wickelgren, I. 1998. The cerebellum: The brain's engine of agility. *Science* 281: 1588–90.

Wilkins, W. K., and J. Wakefield. 1995. Brain evolution and neurolinguistic preconditions. *Behavioral and Brain Sciences* 18: 161–226.

Williams, G. V., and P. S. Goldman-Rakic. 1995. Modulation of memory fields by dopamine D1 receptors in prefrontal cortex. *Nature* 376: 572–575.

Williams, P. L., and R. Warwick. 1980. *Gray's anatomy.* 36th ed. Philadelphia: W. B. Saunders.

Wills, R. H. 1973. *The institutionalized severely retarded.* Springfield, Ill.: Charles C. Thomas.

Wilson, E. O. 1975. *Sociobiology: The new synthesis.* Cambridge, Mass.: Harvard University Press.

Wise, S. P. 1997. Evolution of neuronal activity during conditional motor learning. In *The acquisition of motor behavior in vertebrates,* ed. J. R. Bloedel, T. J. Ebner, and S. P. Wise. Cambridge, Mass.: MIT Press.

Wood, B. A. 1991. *Koobi Fora Research Project.* Vol. 4: *The hominid cranial remains.* Oxford: Clarendon Press.

———1992. Evolution of Australopithecines. In *The Cambridge encyclopedia of human evolution,* ed. S. Jones, R. Martin, and D. Pilbeam. Cambridge: Cambridge University Press. Pp. 231–240.

Wood, B. A., and M. Collard. 1999. The human genus. *Science* 284: 65–71.

Wright, Robert. 1994. *The moral animal.* New York: Random House.

Wulfeck, B. B. 1988. Grammaticality judgments and sentence comprehension in agrammatic aphasia. *Journal of Speech and Hearing Research* 31: 72–81.

Wulfeck, B., and E. Bates. 1991. Differential sensitivity to errors of agreement and word order in Broca's aphasia. *Journal of Cognitive Neuroscience* 3: 258–272.

Wulfeck, B., E. Bates, and R. Capasso. 1991. A cross-linguistic study of grammaticality judgments in Broca's aphasia. *Brain and Language* 41: 311–336.

Xuerob, J. H., B. E. Tomlinson, D. Irving, R. H. Perry, G. Blessed, and E. K. Perry. 1990. Cortical and subcortical pathology in Parkinson's disease: Relationship to Parkinsonian dementia. In *Advances in neurology.* Vol. 53: *Parkinson's disease: Anatomy, pathology, and therapy,* ed. M. B. Streifler, A. D. Korezyn, J. Melamed, and M. B. H. Youdim. New York: Raven Press. Pp. 35–39.

Yamada, J. 1990 *Laura: A case for the modularity of language.* Cambridge, Mass.: MIT Press.

Zatorre, R. J., A. R. Halpern, D. W. Perry, E. Meyer, and A. C. Evans. 1996. Hearing in the mind's ear: A PET investigation of musical imagery and perception. *Journal of Cognitive Neuroscience* 8: 29–46.

Ziles, K., G. Schlaug, M. Matelli, G. Luppino, A. Schleicher, M. Qu, A. Dabringhaus, R. Seitz, and P. E. Roland. 1995. Mapping of human and macaque sensorimotor areas by integrating architectonic, transmitter receptor, MRI, and PET data. *Journal of Anatomy* 187: 515–537.

Zinkin, N. I. 1968. *Mechanisms of speech.* The Hague: Mouton.

Zubrow, E. 1990. The demographic modeling of Neanderthal extinction. In *The human revolution: Behavioral and biological perspectives on the origin of modern humans,* ed. P. Mellars and C. B. Stringer. Vol. 1, pp. 212–231. Edinburgh: Edinburgh University Press.

Zurif, E. B., A. Caramazza, and R. Meyerson. 1972. Grammatical judgments of agrammatic aphasics. *Neuropsychologia* 10: 405–418.

Index

Abstract reasoning/concepts, 2, 77, 80, 90, 95, 99, 116, 153, 154, 158; categories, 113–114
Acoustic system/acoustic(s): signals, 6, 10, 24, 31, 43, 45, 48, 49, 50, 51, 58, 60, 179n12; information, 10, 55, 57–58; energy, 39, 40–41, 42; cues, 41–42, 43, 48, 49, 57, 98, 152, 170n1, 178n7; formant frequencies, 42–43, 51–56; speech and, 45, 47; gender variations in, 53; physical, 54, 57; subphonetic, 76
Acute mountain sickness (AMC), 112
Algorithms, 24, 30, 127, 166; linguistic, 12–13, 14, 159
Alzheimer's disease, 104, 113, 173n5
American Sign Language, 133–134, 135, 152, 163, 178n11; in chimpanzee studies, 131–132. *See also* Sign language
Amphibians, 20–21, 82, 100, 142, 144–145
Anatomical independence, 30
Apes: vocal language, 7; brain volume and size, 100, 150, 167; lack of language and speech, 123, 131, 158, 176n2; linguistic ability, 130, 158; skull configuration, 140; formant frequencies of, 142; supralaryngeal vocal tract, 142; lack of toolmaking technology, 144. *See also* Chimpanzees; Monkeys
Aphasia, 32, 37, 152; syntax comprehension deficits, 3, 175n14; language and lexical deficits, 12, 16, 64, 100, 119, 173n6, 179n4; speech deficits, 41, 94–99; sign language and, 69, 178n11; grammaticality judgments, 76, 95, 171n6, 172n4; basal ganglia as locus of, 94–96, 100–121; syndromes, 96–97; cognitive deficits, 113. *See also* Brain damage; Broca's area; Wernicke's area
Apraxia, oral, 37
Archaeological record: evolution of language and, 124, 142, 152–153; fossils, 125, 128, 142–143, 145, 146, 175n1, 176n5; bipedalism and basal ganglia, 142–143; extinction of Neanderthals, 148–149; genetic discontinuities in, 148–149; of early hominid culture, 152
Ardipithecus ramidus, 142
Articulatory gestures, 118–119, 171n4; of speech motor programs, 108, 151–152; sequencing of, 129; nonlinguistic, 178n11
Associative learning, 11, 22, 26, 57, 89, 164; neural network model, 162–163
Attention deficits, 103, 104
Auditory systems, 10, 38, 179n3; information/signals, 5, 48, 60; perception, 22, 29, 68; functional neural systems and, 33; acoustic energy, 39, 40–41; speech production and, 39; frequencies, 41, 43; voice-onset time and, 58; neural bases of, 63; stimuli, 66, 162; comprehension deficits, 102

Augmented transition network (ATN), 179n4
Australopithecines, 135, 143, 175n1
Australopithecus afarensis, 143
Automatization, 35–36
Axons, 22, 29, 177n5

Baddeley's theory of verbal working memory, 69, 70, 171n4
Basal ganglia: cognition and, 1, 89, 94, 158; language and, 1, 83, 87; motor control function, 1–2, 7, 10, 21, 93–94, 109; as subcortical structure, 1, 7, 10, 16, 33, 80, 81, 84, 85, 100–101, 108–109, 123, 158, 159; sequencing regulation, 4–5, 91–93, 108–109, 112, 116–119, 122, 159; functional language system and, 16, 82, 94, 102–103, 118–119, 123, 143, 158, 159; in animals, 20–21, 85, 153; circuitry, 82, 85–87, 91, 93, 94, 108, 117, 119, 121–123, 153, 164, 165, 169n1, 172n2; function, 82–83, 88; striatal structures, 83, 85, 87, 89, 90, 130, 151, 153, 158; structure of, 83–87, 92, 118–119, 161; computation function, 85, 90, 91, 121, 160; damage to, 85, 99, 109, 118, 120, 122–123, 130, 143, 165, 167; internal and external segments (GPi, GPe), 85, 86, 89, 90, 93; neuronal populations in, 85–86; parallel processing by, 85–86, 93; neurobiological studies of, 87–94; syntax and, 87–88, 121; learned behavior and, 89–91; stereotaxic surgery on, 93–94; aphasia and, 94–96, 100–121; cognitive deficits and, 95, 99–100, 113–116; speech function of, 96–99, 112–113, 131; neurodegenerative diseases and, 102–103; Parkinson's disease and syntax, 103–106; hypoxia and, 109–112; comprehension deficits and, 112–113; verbal working memory and, 116–119; volume and size, 130; bipedalism and, 142–143, 151. *See also* Brain anatomy: subcortical structures
Behavior, 75, 85, 89; neural bases of, 3, 22, 29, 30–32, 61, 66, 68, 109; animal, 4, 8, 66, 161; complex, 4, 22, 31, 35, 66, 82; regulation of, 4, 7, 158, 161, 164; linguistic theory and, 15, 62; derived features of, 17; of hominids, 17; deficits, 22, 32, 83, 99–100, 101, 108, 109, 129, 130; learned, 25, 89–91; visual information and, 33; adaptive, 35; motor equivalence in, 43; cognitive, 80; commonality of human and chimpanzee, 124; genetic bases for, 125, 126–127, 175n1; bound vs. adaptive, 153–154
Bell, Alexander Graham, 45–46, 56
Bickerton, Derek, 126, 127, 134
Biological evolution, 6, 15, 17, 108, 128, 159, 160, 164
Biological fitness, 6, 15, 74–75, 126, 137, 141, 156, 158; motor response and, 1–2; differences in, 149; functional neural systems and, 153
Biological linguistics, 17–18, 165–166, 167
Bipedalism, 156; neural bases of, 7, 33; in chimpanzees, 124, 125; evolution of, 124–125; in hominids, 141, 142–143, 145, 151; basal ganglia and, 142–143
Birds, 144–145, 154–155, 166
Blindness, 27, 66–67
Brain, 4, 85; functional organization, 2, 119, 159, 167; plasticity, 5, 11, 66–69, 81, 83, 152, 157, 161–162, 164, 167, 179n1; circuitry, 9–10, 15–16, 22, 29, 30–33, 35, 36, 61, 62, 64–66, 68, 69, 76, 82, 83, 99, 107, 119, 123, 154, 158, 174n11, 179n1; biological, 13, 15, 25, 70; evolution of, 20, 32, 158–159; theories, 22, 94; cells, 25, 29; computation processes, 26, 32, 62, 151; electrophysiologic recording of activity, 27–29; surgery, 29–30, 172n2; metabolic activity, 30–32, 78, 79–80, 99; language and, 32, 162; of animals, 33, 153, 167; cooperative neural networks, 35; hemispheres, 37, 144–145, 149–150, 169n2; electrical stimulation of, 38–39, 63, 75–76, 95; dictionary in, 61–66, 69, 81, 96; regulation of, 68; species-specific attributes, 131, 154; volume and size, 100, 135–

136, 143, 145–146, 146–147, 150–151; hominid evolution of, 149–151; encephalization quotient (EQ), 150; morphology, 158–159; information flow, 172n1. *See also* Broca's area; Brodmann, Korbinian/Brodmann's areas; Mind-brain theories; Wernicke's area

Brain anatomy, 19; subcortical structures, 1, 2, 5–7, 10, 16, 21, 27, 33–34, 68, 77, 80–83, 89, 93, 100, 106, 113, 119–121, 123, 151, 153, 158, 159; cerebral hemispheres, 3–4, 20–21, 27, 37, 68, 144, 149–150, 169n2; brain-behavior relationships and, 4; cortical areas and maps, 5, 27; animal, 20–21, 28, 29–30; cerebellum, 20, 21, 78, 81, 82, 83, 89, 119–121, 122, 150, 154, 159; in amphibians, 20–21, 82; cerebrum, 20–21; functional neural systems and, 20–21; paleocortex, 20–21; hippocampus, 21; midbrain structures, 21; neuron pathways, 21, 22, 29–30, 34, 38, 68, 162; dendrites and axons, 22, 177n5; synapses, 22; research, 27–32; in monkeys, 28, 33, 34, 83; tracer studies, 29–30; visual cortex, 33, 34, 66–67; premotor cortex, 34, 37, 63, 78, 81, 86, 159; verbal working memory and, 78–79; of rodents, 83, 87; motor control and, 119–121; hemispheres, 144, 149–150, 169n2; planum temporale (PT), 149–150; functional language system and, 154; sensory cortex, 159. *See also* Basal ganglia; Brain damage: to subcortical structures; Cortex; Distributed neural networks; Motor cortex; Neocortex; Prefrontal cortex; Speech production: anatomy for

Brain damage, 31, 86, 174n11, 178n11, 179n4; language deficits, 3, 5, 11–12, 17, 27, 67, 94–99, 102; in children, 5, 67, 68, 69; functional language system and, 5; distributed neural networks and, 11; recovery from, 17; behavioral deficits, 22, 32, 83; lexical retrieval and, 64; outside cortical areas, 64; naming deficits, 64–65, 95; verbal working memory deficits, 79; to cortex, 95, 96; motor control deficits, 101, 152; to subcortical structures, 101, 108, 113–116; effect on sequencing, 108–109; cognitive deficits, 113–116; hemisphere dominance and, 144. *See also* Aphasia; Basal ganglia: damage; Parkinson's disease

Brain-mind-language relationship. *See* Mind-brain theories; Modular theories of mind

Broca, Paul, 7, 22, 23, 32, 94

Broca's area, 4, 28, 114, 158; as seat of language, 2, 7–8, 27, 121, 128, 145–146; damage to, 3, 22; aphasia, 9, 16, 41, 63, 94–99, 101–103, 105, 106, 108, 119, 123, 173n5, 174n11; speech production and, 37; verbal working memory and, 77, 78, 79, 81, 105, 175n13; syndrome, 100, 101; motor control and, 105, 159

Broca-Wernicke theory, 3–4, 22, 37, 64, 83

Brodmann, Korbinian/Brodmann's areas, 27, 28, 38, 63, 86, 114, 175n13

Bunge, Mario, 13, 14

Caplan, David, 72

Cerebellum. *See* Brain anatomy

"Cheater-detector" gene, 126, 127, 128, 155

Chimpanzees: lack of language and speech, 100, 131–133, 136, 150, 177n5; bipedalism, 124, 125; neural capacity, 125; mating patterns, 126; sign language and, 130, 152; syntax and protolangauge, 133–136; vocalization, 136; supralaryngeal vocal tract, 137–138, 177n5; brain volume and size, 143, 145–146, 149–150, 151

Chomsky, Noam, 3, 7, 13, 72, 175n1; theories of syntax, 1, 11, 164; language regulation theory, 8; transformational grammar theory, 12, 147, 163; generative grammar theory, 14; evolutionary model of language, 127–129; algorithmic approach to language, 160; minimalist movement, 166; nativist agenda, 176n1. *See also* Universal Grammar

Cineradiographic studies of speech production, 43, 46, 50–51, 54
Cognition/cognitive ability, 11, 33, 153, 156; basal ganglia and, 1, 10, 89, 94, 158; neural bases of, 2, 17, 80, 83, 120, 152; nonlinguistic, 7, 119; language and, 17, 82, 166; regulation of, 21, 83, 86, 120, 121, 123; motor activity and, 27; verbal working memory and, 70; final-word recall tests of, 71–72, 76, 117, 171n4; in infants, 75; complex, 82; parallel processing and, 83; deficits, 95–96, 99–100, 109, 113–116, 122, 129, 179n6; sequencing and, 109, 143; evolution of, 128–129; hominid, 147, 154; environmental challenges and opportunities and, 166
Color perception, 8, 56, 62, 63, 159, 165
Computer(s), 9, 11, 13, 25; mechanical-biological analogies to the brain, 23–24; processing, 31, 49; speech synthesizers/simulation, 49, 50, 52, 54, 162; sign language, 130; used in chimpanzee language testing, 133
Computerized tomography (CT), 20, 31, 99
Consonants. *See* Speech perception
Cortex: plasticity, 5, 11, 66–69, 83; neuroanatomical structures, 6; language and, 8, 15; feed-forward and -back connections in, 10–11; brain damage and, 11, 27; animal, 20–21; neural pathways, 22, 38, 39; visual, 27, 62, 63; auditory, 38; organization of, 67–68, 171n5; somatosensory, 86; sensorimotor, 90, 172n3; stimulation studies, 170n2
Crelin, Edmund, 176n5
Croft, William, 14–15
Cross-fostering experiments, 132, 133–134
Cytoarchitectonic structures, 27, 28

Darwin, Charles, 19, 126, 127, 128, 138–139, 159; evolutionary theory, 7, 15, 17, 156, 160, 169n1; uniformitarianism theory, 126, 148; genetic variation theory, 140, 165; on struggle for existence, 153; common ancestry theory, 171n3. *See also* Evolution
Deafness and hearing impairment, 45–46, 49, 57–58, 69, 104, 121, 132, 133, 162, 163; sign languages and, 152
Dementia, 103, 104, 113, 173n5
Derived features: evolution of, 2–3, 17, 124, 125, 158; of *Homo sapiens*, 20, 136; of language and linguistic ability, 100, 130, 136, 142, 158; species-specific, 140, 166; of hominids, 143–144, 158
Dialects, 148–149, 162, 178n10
Distinctions in meaning, 37; syntax and, 5, 17, 61, 62, 95, 104, 119; comprehension of, 104, 172n4, 175n14
"Distinctions in Meaning Conveyed by Syntax" test (TMS), 108–109, 117–118, 120
Distributed neural networks, 2, 19, 35, 81, 121, 130, 164; functional neural systems and, 3–7; effect on motor response, 4, 93; damage to, 11, 25–26; computer models of, 22, 91; hidden units in, 25, 26; multilayered, 25, 26; functional language system as, 83; abstract concepts and, 90; syntax and, 163; associative, 179n4. *See also* Neuron(s)/neural mechanisms
DNA, 146
Dopamine: learned behavior and, 90; depletion, 93, 117, 119, 122; in neural circuits, 106–107; levodopa medication, 93, 115–116
Down's syndrome, 131, 152

Electroencephalograms (EEGs), 32, 75, 92
Electrophysiologic studies, 27–29, 32, 33, 34, 67, 79
Elman, Jeffrey, 68, 69, 164
Emotion, 2, 4, 81, 86, 136
Encephalization quotient (EQ), 150
Event-related potentials (ERPs), 31–32, 75, 76
Event-time histograms, 88
Evolution, 74, 166; of functional language system, 1–2, 3, 7, 122, 142–155, 156,

158; of language, 1, 4, 19, 45–46, 124, 125, 127–129, 130–142, 155, 156; of derived features, 2–3, 17, 124, 125, 158; biological, 6, 15, 17, 108, 128, 159, 160, 164; brain, 6, 20, 158–159; lineages, 100; of behavior, 125; psychological, 125–130; of syntax, 126, 128; of motor control, 128; of speech, 128, 142, 151, 154, 155; ontogenetic, 140; "Eve" hypothesis, 146, 171n3; multiregional theory, 146; out-of-Africa theory, 146; of modern human beings, 146–148; of bipedalism, 151; cognitive science and, 158–159; hominid, 175n1; of supralaryngeal vocal tract, 176n5
Eye-tracking data, 73

Feed-forward and -back connections, 10–11
Final-word recall tests, 71–72, 76, 117, 171n4
Fingers. *See* Hand movement
Fodor, J., 8, 9–10, 64
Formant frequencies, 42–44, 45, 154–155, 179n12; in children, 44, 51; patterns of, 47, 49–50, 51–57, 106, 162–164; gender variations in, 53; anatomy and, 54, 170n2; for stop consonants, 56, 57, 98, 106, 117–118, 162–163; associative learning and, 57; speech production and, 97, 102; modulation of, 136; in monkeys and apes, 142; syllable-onset, 162–164. *See also* Speech production
Functional language system (FLS), 15, 37, 167; evolution of, 1–2, 3, 7, 122, 142–155, 156, 158; regulatory function of, 1, 6; neural bases of, 2, 6, 7, 16, 17, 82, 83, 94, 101, 121, 153, 154, 160; in *Homo sapiens*, 33; speech and, 41, 45, 155; as distributed neural network, 61, 83, 157; verbal working memory and, 70; circuitry, 81, 158, 167; basal ganglia and, 102–103, 118–119, 123, 143, 158, 159; bipedalism and, 143–144, 151; manual dexterity and, 143–144, 151–153; brain volume and size and, 145–146; hominid vs. ape brains and, 149–151; hominid language and, 151–153; sign language and, 151–153; bound vs. adaptive behavior, 153–154; talking birds and, 154–155; anatomy of, 158, 161; computation function, 158
Functional magnetic resonance imaging (fMRI), 75, 77, 79, 80, 113; noninvasive imaging studies, 30–32; motor cortex studies, 67–68
Functional neural systems (FNS), 153, 157, 158, 160; distributed neural networks and, 3–7; modularity and, 7–11; historical background, 19, 20–32; brain anatomy and, 20–21; in monkeys, 29, 33, 79; for objects close to the eye, 29, 33, 34; for motor control and vision, 32–36
Fundamental frequency (F0), 40, 48–49, 53, 59–60, 107, 142, 178n7. *See also* Phonation/phonetics

Gardner, Alan, 131–132, 133–134
Gardner, Beatrix, 131–132, 133–134
Genetics/gene(s), 68, 166; molecular, 69; language and, 75, 129–130, 146, 167; deficits, 123; commonality of human and chimpanzee, 124; behavior and, 125; of neural mechanisms, 125; "cheater-detector," 126, 127, 128, 155; as dating technique, 146; archaeological record and, 148–149; motor control and, 164; variations in, 164–165
Geschwind, N., 22, 23
Goldstein, Kurt, 99
Goodall, Jane, 136
Grammar, 15, 135, 152, 173n4; core, 12, 14–15, 171n3; generative, 12, 160; rules, 12–13, 14, 127, 163; transformational, 12, 147, 163; ungrammatical formations, 12, 76–77, 95; intuitive, 14, 18; agrammatical speech, 38, 95, 171n6, 172n4; neural bases of, 69; verbal working memory and, 73–74, 76–77, 78, 105, 172n7; paragrammatism, 96; children's acquisition of, 127, 132; vocabulary size

Grammar *(continued)*
and, 131; matrix, 179n4. *See also* Universal Grammar
Gross, Charles, 33, 34

Handedness, 68, 145
Hand movement: neural bases of, 33, 81; motor control of, 35, 63, 65, 160; fingers, 67–68, 160; manual dexterity, 143–144, 151–153
Haskins Laboratories, 43, 48, 49
Hearing. *See* Auditory systems; Deafness and hearing impairment
Hebb's theory of synaptic modification, 22, 25, 90
High-altitude studies, 109–112
Holloway, Ralph, 146
Hominid evolution, 175n1, 176n5; anatomy and bipedal locomotion, 124–125, 151; functional language system and, 146–148, 152, 154, 156; of the brain, 149–151
Hominids, 17; speech capability, 7; brain volume and size, 128, 143, 145, 150; syntactic ability, 135; bipedalism, 141, 142–143, 145, 151; supralaryngeal vocal tract, 142; derived features, 143–144, 158; tools/toolmaking technology, 143–144, 145; fossils, 145; linguistic ability, 145, 147; extinction, 158; lexical and syntactic ability, 158. *See also Homo sapiens*
Homo erectus, 7, 128, 136, 141, 145, 146, 178n8
Homo ergaster, 145, 146
Homo habilis, 128, 145, 146
Homo rudolfensis, 145
Homo sapiens, 7, 135, 141, 147, 154, 155; derived features, 20, 136. *See also* Hominids
Huntington's disease, 103
Hypobaric chamber tests, 112
Hypoxia, 119, 120, 123; Mount Everest study, 109–112, 123, 174n12

Imaging systems and studies, 71, 100–101, 159, 167, 175n13, 178n11; noninvasive, 30–32; for speech production and perception, 37, 46; mental, 38; for patterns, 63; brain, 66; vision systems and, 67. *See also* Functional magnetic resonance imaging (fMRI); Magnetic resonance imaging (MRI)
Imitation, 11
Information, 4; sensory, 2, 82, 157, 158; pragmatic, 5, 24–25, 58, 62, 75, 76, 134, 157; acoustic, 10, 57–58; flow and exchange, 16; semantic, 24–25, 75–76, 106; top-down, 24; lexical, 58, 78; coding, 62, 157, 161; processing, 71, 85; nonsyntactic, 72, 73, 74; contextual, 75; linguistic, 75, 82, 152; situational, 75; syntactic, 75, 127; phonetic, 154, 173n9; conceptual, 157, 158; visual, 157
Inheritance, soft, 128, 129
Initial thinking time, 115–116
Innateness, 69, 125, 179n3; of language, 1, 2, 5, 9, 127, 130, 166; of syntactic ability, 1, 13, 68; of Universal Grammar, 5, 13, 127, 162, 163; of knowledge, 13, 162, 163, 170n3; of grooming behavior, 87–88; of manual motor control, 92–93; of speech perception, 141–142; of preferences, 175n1

Jackendoff, Ray, 12, 160
Jakobson, Roman, 47
Just and Carpenter memory models, 71, 72, 73–74

Kagan, Jerome, 31, 125
Keller, Helen, 152
Knowledge: storage of, 2; linguistic, 5, 8, 157; innateness of, 13, 162, 163, 170n3; semantic, 61, 62, 95; real-world, 62, 64, 81; conceptual, 64; object, 66; phonological, 79; syntactic, 161
Krakauer, John, 112

Lamarck, Jean Baptiste, 128, 129
Language: evolution, 1, 4, 19, 45–46, 124, 125, 127–129, 130–142, 155; innateness,

1, 2, 5, 9, 127, 130, 166; neural bases, 1, 2, 7–8, 15–17, 19, 20, 22, 23, 32, 37, 61, 81, 83, 87, 100, 112, 120, 121, 123, 130, 131, 144–146, 147, 152, 155, 166, 167, 178n11; manual systems and signs, 2–3, 6, 130; regulation, 2, 6, 11, 21, 27, 82, 94, 121, 157, 164; spoken, 2, 22, 24, 82; biological bases, 3, 17, 74–75, 130; deficits, 3, 12, 22, 32, 64, 83, 94–99, 96, 101, 116, 119, 165; expressive, 3, 96; acquisition, 5–6, 27, 130–131; coding, 5, 161; critical periods, 5–6; lack of, in animals, 8, 16, 32, 100, 123, 128, 131–133, 136, 150, 158, 176n2, 177n5; processing, 8, 10, 67, 83; comprehension, 10, 12, 24, 77, 95, 96, 100, 116; neuroanatomical structures and, 11, 81; retention of, after brain damage, 11; knowledge of, 13–14; sound patterns of, 47; preservation, 67; speech and, 70, 136; capacity and working memory, 72; contextual information, 75; development in infants, 75; morphology, 75; vocal imitation, 75; word production, 75; as derived feature, 100, 158; cognition and, 127–128, 166; preadaptive bases for, 128; vs. communication in primates, 128; genetic bases of, 130, 146; syntax and protolanguage in chimpanzees, 133–136, 155; inflected, 135, 175n14; antiquity of, 136–142; hominid, 145, 146–148, 151–153, 156; dialects, 148–149, 162; studies and public policy, 166–167; recovery in aphasic patients, 179n4. *See also* Aphasia; Functional language system; Lexical ability; Linguistic ability; Speech

Laryngeal function. *See* Voice-onset time (VOT)

Learning: language, 12–13, 161–162; rule-based, 25, 89, 90; behavioral, 89–91; supervised, 90–91; motor, 119

Levodopa treatment, 93, 115–116. *See also* Dopamine

Lexical ability, 7, 10; access and retrieval, 16–17, 37, 61, 62, 63, 76, 109, 174n9; brain damage and, 64; phonation and, 64; verb/noun, 64; basal ganglia and, 83; in apes, 158; "on-line" test of, 172n4

Lexicon, 8, 9, 127, 157, 174n9; evolution of, 61; neural bases of, 62; phonetic addresses in, 70; information coded in, 74, 78; vocabulary size, 128, 130, 131, 132, 135; syntax and, 135

Liberman, Alvin, 43, 48, 57, 58

Lichtheim, L., 22, 38

Lichtheim-Geschwind theory, 3–4, 15, 145–156

Linguistic ability, 7, 8, 10, 32, 87, 128, 157, 163; neural bases of, 3, 6, 76, 77, 100, 125, 149–150, 158, 159; in children, 11, 27, 131, 135, 148, 149, 162, 179n6; grammar and, 12–13, 76; genetic bases for, 13, 126, 129–130; prosody and, 58–60; acoustic systems and, 60; deficits, 63, 129–130, 150, 165, 179n6, 180n6; sensitive periods, 66–69, 162, 179n1; brain damage and, 67, 68, 69, 102; variations in, 74, 75; syntax and, 87; as derived feature, 100, 130, 136, 142, 158; sequencing deficits, 105; evolution of, 127–129, 156; innateness of, 127; species-specific, 127, 131, 154; sudden mutation as basis of, 127–128; capacity limitation, 130–131; of chimpanzees, 131–133; mental retardation and, 131; dissociated from speech production, 133; of hominids, 145, 147, 154; of Neanderthals, 176n5. *See also* Broca's area; Brodmann, Korbinian/Brodmann's areas; Wernicke's area

Linguistic theory, 22, 59, 72, 76, 129, 159, 160, 172n4; mind-brain theories, 8–9, 23–25, 45, 94, 159–160; neophrenological, 8, 19, 23, 30–31, 128, 167; plasticity of neuroanatomical structures, 11, 81; syntax in, 11–12, 78, 161; algorithmic solutions, 12–13, 14, 159; theories of data, 13–15, 18; competence/performance distinction, 14–15, 172n7; neural network basis, 16; biological, 17–18, 165–166, 167; mechanical-biological

Linguistic theory *(continued)*
analogies, 23–24; modular, 24, 64, 167; rules vs. representation, 26; nativistic, 74; interactive-activation models, 78; sudden mutation as basis of linguistic ability, 127–128; construction grammar, 135; minimalist (Chomskian), 135; locationist, 167
Lip-reading, 57

Magnetic resonance imaging (MRI), 20, 30, 31, 35, 102, 109, 130, 150, 177n5
Mayr, Ernst, 17, 19, 74, 166
McGurk effect, 57
Mellars, Paul, 147
Memory, 109; short- and long-term, 4, 69, 173n9; distributed neural networks and, 22, 25; local, 26; computation function, 69, 70, 81; storage function, 69, 70; visuospatial, 70–71; capacity, 71, 72; spatial, 89; spans in children, 113; traces, 159, 171n4. *See also* Verbal working memory
Mesulam, M. M., 4, 16, 62
Mind-brain theories, 8–9, 23–25, 45, 94, 159–160
Modularity, 2, 33, 34, 61, 108; functional neural systems and, 7–11; of syntax, 11, 72–75; of computers, 24; in linguistic theory, 24, 64, 167; somatopic, 35; of speech, 58, 170n3; sequencing and, 88; of formant frequencies, 136
Modular theories of mind, 2, 7, 8, 9–10, 11, 24, 159
Mollusks, 2, 25, 153
Monkeys, 4; acoustic ability, 10; hand-eye motor control, 17, 33; brain anatomy, 28, 33, 34, 35, 71, 83, 106, 113, 125, 150, 153; macaque, 28, 33, 150, 170n2; functional neural systems, 29, 33, 79; sensory perception, 33–34; visuospatial working memory, 70–71; associative learning, 89–90; spatial working memory, 89; sequencing experiments, 92; brain damage, 93; speech production, 107; formant frequencies, 142; supralaryngeal vocal tract, 142
Montreal Neurological Institute, 37
Morphemes, 175n14
Morphology, 17, 51, 75, 120, 128, 152, 172n4; rules, 11, 164; skeletal, 140, 148, 176n5; of human brain, 158–159, 162; of verbs, 163
Morphophonemics, 134
Motion perception, 63, 64
Motor control, 157; basal ganglia and, 1–2, 7, 21, 93–94, 109; environmental challenges and opportunities, 1, 7, 17, 158; linguistic ability and, 2; neural bases of, 2, 17, 22, 27, 38, 81, 83, 89, 119–121, 122, 128, 129, 143, 152–153, 160–161, 179n5; evolution of, 3, 128, 129; goal-directed, 4, 82, 90; regulation of, 4, 86, 121, 122, 158–159, 160, 178n11; hand movement, 5, 17, 33, 34, 79, 101, 143–144; of speech and speech production, 6, 38, 43, 44–45, 50, 78, 79; manual, 7, 10, 27, 79, 92–93, 95, 102, 105, 143–144, 151–153, 156; functional neural systems and, 32–36; body and muscles, 34–35, 90; programs (MCPs), 35–36, 44, 82, 86, 107, 108, 143, 161; deficits, 37, 95, 101, 102, 103, 115, 118–119, 152, 174n9; lexical retrieval and, 64; sequencing, 82, 91, 92, 100, 103, 118, 122, 123, 143; parallel processing and, 83; brain circuitry, 85–87; learned behavior and, 89–91; innateness of, 92–93; spatial cues, 92; temporal cues, 92; compensatory, 103–104; preadaptive, 143; submovements, 153–154; genetics and, 164; syntax and, 175n15
Motor cortex, 86, 159; electrical stimulation of, 21, 22, 32; primary, 27, 34–35, 36, 62; in monkeys, 34, 35; speech production and, 37; functional magnetic resonance imaging of, 67–68; matrisomes, 90
Motor equivalence, 39, 43–45, 50
Movement-related potentials (MRPs), 91, 92

Müller, Johannes, 39, 42, 47, 56
Mutism. *See* Deafness and hearing impairment

Naming of objects and animals, 38–39, 66, 71, 81, 103, 132, 170n2, 173n6, 174n9; neural bases of, 33; deficits, 62–63, 64–65, 95, 98
Natural selection, 1–2, 5, 7, 15, 126, 128, 141, 156, 158
Neanderthals, 135; speech capability, 7, 141; supralaryngeal vocal tract, 139–140, 177n6, 178n10; skeletal anatomy, 140, 148; brain volume and size, 146–147; cultural borrowing by, 147–148; linguistic ability, 147; extinction of, 148–149
Nearey, Terrance, 43, 46, 47, 50–51, 54–55
Neocortex, 1, 2, 4, 77, 84; language and, 7, 100, 121; animal, 20; damage to, 22; speech production and, 37; verbal working memory and, 81; in monkeys, 125, 136; size of, 151
Neologisms, 96
Neophrenological theories, 8, 19, 23, 30–31, 128, 167
Neuroanatomical structures, 4, 15; functional language system and, 6, 7, 16, 121, 157–158, 160; computation function, 11, 24, 26, 81, 82; genetically specified, 11; plasticity of, 11, 81; for speech and language, 11, 62, 69, 70, 81, 154; mapping of, 16, 29–30; motor control and, 17, 27; animal, 20–21, 30; acoustic signals and, 31; coding of words and, 63; damage to, 86, 101, 178n11. *See also* Brain anatomy
Neurobiology, 3, 18; studies and data, 2, 7, 13, 17, 77, 79, 127, 149; verbal working memory, 77–81; cognition and, 83; basal ganglia operations, 87–94, 121; neural bases of language, 152
Neurodegenerative diseases, 102–103
Neuron(s)/neural mechanisms: motor control and, 1–2; plasticity, 5, 11, 66–69, 81; electrophysiologic techniques to map, 6, 27–29; mapping of circuits, 6, 8, 16, 29–30; structure of, 20, 21–22, 27, 61; pathways, 21, 22, 29–30, 34, 38, 68, 162; electrochemical communications between, 28–29; putamental, 33–34; cortical, 34–35; visual, 34; regulation of speech, 37–39; firing patterns, 87–88. *See also* Distributed neural networks
Neuronal populations, 5, 63, 121, 157–158; connections among, 2, 22; in animal brains, 4, 30; in basal ganglia, 85–86; regulation of movement, 93
Neurophysiology, 25, 62; models and data, 4, 23–24, 63, 66, 83, 117; vision studies, 33; language studies, 128–129
Noise: turbulent, 39, 41, 46, 53; sources, 41, 42, 45, 56; in distributed neural networks, 90
Number(s): recall, 70, 77; number-span-backward and -forward tests, 116, 118, 120, 174n12

Object identification. *See* Naming of objects and animals
Odd-Man-Out test, 109, 113, 116, 117–118, 120, 174n12
Ojemann, George, 29, 38, 63
Olduvai Gorge, Tanzania, 143–144, 147
Olfactory perception, 25, 29
On the Origin of Species (Darwin), 17, 19
Ontogenetic evolution, 140, 175n15
Orangutans, 136, 150. *See also* Chimpanzees; Monkeys
Orofacial movements, 38, 129

Paleolithic era, 135, 147
Paleoneurology, 145–146
Palmer, Jeffrey, 141
Parallel processing, 25, 58, 71, 83, 85–86, 90, 93
Parkinson's disease (PD), 17, 102; speech deficits, 41, 103, 108, 172n5; sequencing deficits, 91, 92, 94, 116, 119; cause of,

Parkinson's disease *(continued)*
93; dopamine depletion, 93, 117, 119, 122; cognitive deficits, 103, 113, 116, 118, 120, 122–123; comprehension deficits, 103–104, 105, 117, 118, 119, 174n10; syntax deficits, 103–106, 175n14; effect on grammaticality judgments, 105; voice-onset time deficits, 106, 107, 110; motor control deficits, 109, 111, 112, 115, 174n9; planning deficits, 114; verbal working memory and sequencing in, 116–119; damage to cerebellum, 119; symptoms, 122, 143; semantic deficits, 174n9; hypophonia, 174n11
Passive transformational rule, 12, 14
Pavlov, Ivan, 25
Performance effects, 14, 172n7
Personality, 74–75
Phenotypes, 38, 69, 74
Phonation/phonetics, 6, 8, 9, 10, 24, 41, 62, 98, 155, 174n9; periodic, 39, 174n11; fundamental frequency of, 40, 48–49, 53, 59–60, 107, 142, 178n7; articulatory vs. auditory, 43, 45–48, 50, 56–58; coding, 43, 171n4; information, 57–58; rehearsal mechanism, 61, 70, 77, 78, 79, 112–113, 123, 171n4; lexical retrieval and, 64; in verbal working memory, 79; phonological disorders, 96; dysarthia, 98, 103, 106; formant frequencies, 107; associations, 121; morphophonemics, 134; hominid evolution and, 148–149
Phrenology, 3, 8. *See also* Neophrenological theories
Phylogenetics, 25, 144
Piatelli-Palmarini, Massimo, 165, 180n7
Pinker, Steven, 2, 3–4, 129, 163, 175n1
Planning, 2, 77, 80, 89, 96, 97, 144; deficits, 37, 114
Plasticity. *See* Brain: plasticity; Neuron(s)/neural mechanisms: plasticity
Pleistocene era, 126, 175n1
Positron emission tomography (PET), 30, 31–32, 37, 62, 63, 65, 67, 99, 119, 123; for verbal working memory testing, 77–79, 81
Prefrontal cortex, 81, 89, 150, 153, 159; verbal working memory and, 71, 80; linguistic ability and, 77; cognition and, 80, 83; sequencing and, 92; damage to, 99; size of, 151; functional language system and, 154
Premotor cortex. *See* Brain anatomy
Primates, 67, 136; brain anatomy, 83, 92, 93; associative learning, 89, 90; lack of speech, 128; skull configuration, 140; nonhuman, 142, 154, 159, 172n2
Problem-solving, 5, 114–116
Progressive supranuclear palsy (PSP), 102–103
Project Washoe, 131–132, 133
Prosody, 58–60
Psychoacoustic experiments, 51–52, 54, 59
Psycholinguistic theory, 10, 14, 24, 78
Psychology, evolutionary, 125–130
Putamen. *See* Brain anatomy: subcortical structures

Radioactive tracers, 29–30
Radiographic studies of speech production, 43, 46, 47, 50–51, 139, 141, 177n5
Rats. *See* Rodents
Reading, 38, 150, 179n6
Reading-span tests, 71–72, 74
Reptiles, 20–21, 100
Retardation, 131
Rhode Island Test of Language Structure (RITLS), 104, 106, 110, 111, 112, 116
Rodents: brain anatomy, 83, 87; grooming patterns, 87–88, 92, 153

Saturation effect, 53
Saussure, F. de, 13
Segregation (anatomical independence), 30
Semantic(s): information, 61, 62, 71, 75; verbal working memory and, 70; cues, 73; sentence structure and, 73–74; word substitutions, 96; noun-verb association, 119–120; neural bases of, 159; deficits, 172n4, 174n9; priming effects, 173n9

Sensory systems, 2, 21, 82, 85, 157; taste, 25; tactile, 27, 29, 33, 34, 63, 67–68, 162. *See also* Auditory systems; Vision/vision systems

Sentence(s), 59, 157, 160; structure, 12, 14, 17, 71–73, 76, 79, 80, 81, 104–105, 109, 117; comprehension, 70, 71, 75, 76, 79–80, 83, 112, 120, 121, 158, 172n4; center-embedded, 74, 78, 116, 172n7; processing, 78; complex, 104; comprehension deficits, 104–105, 109, 112–113, 116–119, 171n6, 174n10; active-voice, 109; noun-verb association, 119–120

Sequencing, 153, 156; basal ganglia and, 4–5, 91–93, 108–109, 122, 159; modularity of, 11, 88; verbal working memory and, 70, 116–119; motor control and, 82, 87, 88, 103, 107, 118, 143; deficits, 91, 92, 94, 100, 102, 105–109, 116–120, 122, 123, 129–130, 174n11; regulation of, 91–93, 122; of voice-onset time, 108; cognition and, 109, 117, 143; in speech production, 120–121; in cerebellum, 122; of articulation, 129; family KE study, 129–130

Shapes, 8, 62, 63

Sign language, 69; in chimpanzee studies, 130, 131–132, 152; manual, 151–153, 162. *See also* American Sign Language

Singer, Wolf, 68

Sound, 136; patterns, 2, 6, 42–43, 62, 81, 170n1; localization of, 10, 58; changes, 45, 46; response to, 89–90. *See also* Phonation/phonetics

Space-time relationships, 64

Specific language impairment (SLI), 179n6

Speech, 3, 8, 24, 61, 70; motor control and, 6, 78, 79, 100, 122, 156; silent, 6, 77; neural bases of, 10, 35, 122, 131, 154, 155, 167; deficits, 22, 102; inner, 38, 130, 157; sounds, 39, 45, 47, 48, 49, 57, 60, 64, 76, 98, 107, 118, 125, 170n4, 179n12; pitch, 40, 48–49; patterns, 42–43, 44, 51–53; rates, 43, 112–113, 157; visible, 46; mode, 48, 49–50, 58; synthesizers, 49, 50, 52, 54, 57, 133; transmission coding, 49; articulation, 55, 56–58; signals, 55, 57, 69; intelligibility, 57–58; fluency, 58–59, 131; regulation, 82, 83, 123, 148, 154, 158; formant frequencies, 97; dysarthia, 98, 103, 106; sequencing, 98, 122, 123; articulatory gestures, 108, 118–119, 151–152; lack of, in animals, 123; evolution of, 128, 142, 151, 154, 155; as derived feature, 136, 158; "motherese," 136; supralaryngeal vocal tract and, 141; voluntary, 152, 153, 154; functional language system and, 155; vocal, 157; modularity, 170n3; sine-wave equivalents, 179n12. *See also* Language

Speech perception, 6, 8, 10; functional magnetic resonance imaging for, 30; functional language system and, 37; neural bases of, 37–39, 62, 141–142; of consonant-vowel (CV) segments, 38, 49, 52–53, 58, 112; motor theory of, 38, 43, 48–51, 58; by speech sound, 47–48; vocal tract normalization and, 51–56, 139; "naturalness" judgments, 54, 55–56; of consonants, 56, 57, 58; McGurk effect, 57; articulatory gestures, 57–58, 60; supralaryngeal vocal tract and, 57, 136–137, 141, 176n5; duplex, 58; modularity, 58; verbal working memory and, 70; innateness of, 141–142; genetics and, 164

Speech production, 6, 7, 10, 76, 175n15; anatomy for, 3, 5, 38, 39, 40, 42–48, 53, 56, 58–60, 97, 136–142, 155, 166; deficits, 3, 16, 95, 96–99, 101, 108, 109, 130; neural bases of, 23, 37–39, 69, 70, 78, 123, 174n9; functional language system and, 37; motor equivalence in, 39; phonation, 39; physiology of, 39–45, 60; source-filter theory, 39, 47, 155; segmental sounds, 42; radiographic studies of, 43, 46, 47, 50; articulatory and auditory information, 45–48, 50, 51, 56–58, 60, 97, 152; internalized knowledge of, 49; vocal tract normalization, 51–56, 139; body size and, 53; place of articula-

Speech production *(continued)*
tion, 56–57, 110, 111; visual information for, 57–58; prosody, 58–60; lung volumes, 59–60; verbal working memory and, 70; formant frequencies and, 97, 102; sequencing in, 98, 120–121; in monkeys, 107; regulation of, 116, 120, 174n9; dissociated from linguistic ability, 133; hominid evolution of, 152–153; supralaryngeal vocal tract and, 176n5. *See also* Formant frequencies;Voice-onset time
Striatum. *See* Basal ganglia: striatal structures
Strokes, 12, 22, 101–102, 121
Subcortical structures. *See* Basal ganglia; Brain anatomy: subcortical structures
Subtractive technique for imaging, 30–31, 79
Supralaryngeal vocal tract (SVT), 39, 40, 41–43, 46, 47, 50; formant frequencies and, 51, 97; normalization, 51–56, 139, 170n2; size, 51, 54, 55–56, 142, 155; place of articulation and, 56–57, 110, 111; speech production deficits and, 98; neural bases of, 107–108; speech perception and, 136–137; in chimpanzees, 137–138; configuration, 138–139, 140; of Neanderthals, 139–140, 176n5, 177n6; reconstruction experiment, 139–142; hominid evolution and, 148; filter function of, 155; evolution of, 176n5
Swallowing, 56, 93, 137, 148, 178n6
Synaptic weights, 22, 25, 26, 164
Syntax, 2, 7, 59, 101, 162; innateness of, 1, 13, 68; effect of aphasia on, 3, 16; distinctions in meaning, 5, 17, 61, 62, 95, 104, 119; regulation of, 6, 123; neural bases of, 8, 122, 127, 158, 159; rules, 8, 11, 160, 164; brain regulation of, 9; basal ganglia and, 10, 87–88, 121; comprehension in children, 11, 17, 130–131, 135, 163; linguistic theory and, 11–12, 78, 161; modularity of, 11, 72–75; Universal Grammar and, 11–12; acquisition of, 13; comprehension deficits, 17, 103–104, 122, 171n6; complex, 61, 80, 81, 95, 103, 104, 112–113, 116, 156, 158, 171n6; syntactic information, 62, 71, 72, 74, 75, 127, 161; verbal working memory and, 70; final-word recall tests, 71–72, 76, 117, 171n4; processing, 71–72, 75–76, 78, 79; comprehension, 72, 122, 123, 130, 173n7, 175n15; computation of, 72, 73, 74; parsing, 72–73, 78, 79; cues, 74; sequencing of, 88; Parkinson's disease and, 103–106; error rates, 106; evolution of, 126, 128; capacity limitations on apes and children, 130–131; comprehension in apes, 133–136, 158; of hominids, 135; lexicon and, 135; units of, 142; simple, 156; distributed neural networks and, 163; deficits, 165, 172n4, 173n8, 175n14; motor control and, 175n15

Tactile perception, 27, 29, 33, 34, 63, 67–68, 162
Tallel, Paula, 179–180n6
Temporal sensitivity, 32, 58, 92
Thalamus. *See* Brain anatomy: subcortical structures
Thought, 94, 130; neural bases of, 89, 123, 167; symbolic, 99. *See also* Mind-brain theories
Throwing ability, 128–129
Tools/toolmaking technology, 128, 142, 143–144, 145, 152, 175n1; core and flake technique, 147; Mousterian theory of, 147. *See also* Archaeological record
"Tower of London" test, 114–116
Tracer systems, 32, 67, 89, 90, 113, 167
Twins, identical, 31, 75

Ungerleider, Leslie, 66
Uniformitarianism theory, 126, 148
Universal Grammar (UG), 14, 87, 129–130; innateness of, 5, 13, 127, 162, 163; syntax and, 11–12; natural selection and, 15; distributed representation of, 69; genetic bases of, 126, 146, 164–165; evolution of, 128; neural bases of, 128, 149

Variation, 66–69
Verbal dyspraxia, 129
Verbal Fluency test, 116, 120
Verbal working memory, 6, 69, 157; grammaticality judgments, 7, 76–77, 78, 105, 172nn4; phonetic rehearsal mechanism, 61, 70, 77, 78, 79, 112–113, 116, 118, 123, 171n4, 173–174n9; integration of semantic, pragmatic, and syntactic information, 62, 75, 78, 81; neural bases of, 62, 77, 79–80, 81; cognition and, 70; computation function, 70; executive control mechanism, 70, 77, 80, 89, 116–117, 121; functional language system and, 70; sequencing, 70, 116–119; capacity limits, 71–74, 76, 77, 113, 116, 118; evolution, 71; final-word recall tests, 71–72, 76, 117, 171n4; processing, 71, 104; nonsyntactic information and, 72, 73, 74; neurobiological bases of, 77–81, 79; brain anatomy and, 78–79, 175n13; deficits, 79, 80, 105, 109; bilingual ability, 81; cognitive tests for, 116; span, 116–118, 119, 120, 122, 174n12. *See also* Memory
Vision/vision systems, 5, 8, 165; neural bases of, 4, 27, 33, 34, 62, 63, 66–67, 152; binocular, 5; mental imagery, 27, 38; motor activity and, 27; perception, 29, 33–34, 63; functional neural systems and, 32–36; space representation, 33; stimuli, 34, 66–67, 162; signals, 69; visuospatial inputs, 69, 70–71; in animals, 162. *See also* Imaging systems and studies
Visual working memory, 109, 116–117
Vocabulary. *See* Lexicon
Vocal tract, 24. *See also* supralaryngeal vocal tract (SVT)
Voice-onset time (VOT), 56, 58; deficits, 41, 98, 106–108, 120, 174n10; sequencing, 102, 105–107, 108, 120, 174n11; overlap, 106, 107, 110, 111, 112, 116, 118, 120, 122, 123, 173n8; stop-consonant, 110, 111; at high altitude, 112; acoustic cues and, 170n1; size/length, 170n1; categorical perception of, 179n3
Voicing. *See* Phonation
Vowel(s), 106; formant patterns, 51–56, 139; spectral-peak, 139, 155. *See also* Formant frequencies

Wernicke's area, 2, 3, 4, 11, 22, 39, 121, 149, 158, 159; verbal working memory and, 77, 79, 80, 81; aphasia, 96, 97, 101–102, 173n9; as seat of language, 128, 145–146
Wilson, E. O., 125
Wisconsin Card Sorting Task, 113, 117
Word(s), 2, 128; -finding deficits (anomia), 3, 63, 95, 103, 117; coding in, 5, 6, 63, 157; information, 24, 157; syllabic structure of, 26; interpretation/comprehension, 31; spoken, 32, 37, 133; stressed, 58–59, 112; meanings, 61–62, 159; recall tests, 71–72, 76, 117, 171n4, 174n9; inanimate, 73, 74; generation/production, 75, 81, 119–120, 133; "empty," 96; neologisms, 96, 102; substitutions, 102; order, 134, 175n14; grammatical function of, 135; length, 171n4; phonologic representation of, 171n4

Yerkes Language Research Center study, 132–133, 134